362.2. LLO

KT-154-591

£54-99.

Vocational Rehabilitation
and Mental Health

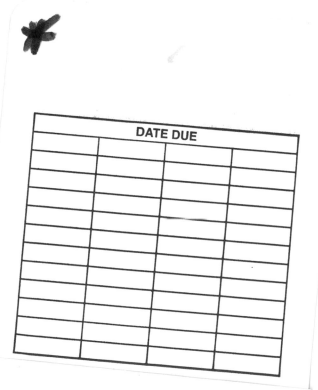

DATE DUE			

TEES, ESK & WEAR VALLEYS
NHS FOUNDATION TRUST
INGLEWOOD LIBRARY
LANCHESTER ROAD HOSPITAL
DURHAM

DEMCO

Vocational Rehabilitation and Mental Health

Edited by

Chris Lloyd

School of Population Health
The University of Queensland and the Queensland and
the Queensland Centre for Mental Health Research
Australia

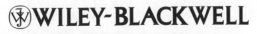

A John Wiley & Sons, Ltd., Publication

This edition first published 2010
© 2010 Blackwell Publishing Ltd
Chapter 8 © 2007 British Journal of Occupational Therapy

Blackwell Publishing was acquired by John Wiley & Sons in February 2007. Blackwell's publishing programme has been merged with Wiley's global Scientific, Technical, and Medical business to form Wiley-Blackwell.

Registered office
John Wiley & Sons Ltd, The Atrium, Southern Gate, Chichester, West Sussex, PO19 8SQ, United Kingdom

Editorial offices
9600 Garsington Road, Oxford, OX4 2DQ, United Kingdom
2121 State Avenue, Ames, Iowa 50014-8300, USA

For details of our global editorial offices, for customer services and for information about how to apply for permission to reuse the copyright material in this book please see our website at www.wiley.com/wiley-blackwell.

The right of the author to be identified as the author of this work has been asserted in accordance with the UK Copyright, Designs and Patents Act 1988.

All rights reserved. No part of this publication may be reproduced, stored in a retrieval system, or transmitted, in any form or by any means, electronic, mechanical, photocopying, recording or otherwise, except as permitted by the UK Copyright, Designs and Patents Act 1988, without the prior permission of the publisher.

Wiley also publishes its books in a variety of electronic formats. Some content that appears in print may not be available in electronic books.

Designations used by companies to distinguish their products are often claimed as trademarks. All brand names and product names used in this book are trade names, service marks, trademarks or registered trademarks of their respective owners. The publisher is not associated with any product or vendor mentioned in this book. This publication is designed to provide accurate and authoritative information in regard to the subject matter covered. It is sold on the understanding that the publisher is not engaged in rendering professional services. If professional advice or other expert assistance is required, the services of a competent professional should be sought.

Library of Congress Cataloging-in-Publication Data

Vocational rehabilitation and mental health / [edited by] Chris Lloyd.
    p. ; cm.
  Includes bibliographical references and index.
  ISBN 978-1-4051-9249-1 (pbk. : alk. paper)
1. People with mental disabilities–Rehabilitation.   2. People with mental disabilities–Employment.
3. Occupational therapy.   I. Lloyd, Chris, 1954–
[DNLM: 1. Mental Disorders–rehabilitation.   2. Rehabilitation, Vocational.   3. Employment–psychology. HV 3005 V872 2010]
  HV3005.V63 2010
  362.2–dc22

                                                                                              2009037335

A catalogue record for this book is available from the British Library.

Set in 10.5/13 pt Sabon by Aptara® Inc., New Delhi, India
Printed and bound in Malaysia by Vivar Printing Sdn Bhd

1   2010

CONTENTS

CONTRIBUTORS

Patrick W. Corrigan, Psy D, is Professor and Associate Dean for Research at the Institute of Psychology, Illinois Institute of Technology in Chicago. For the past 25 years, he has worked to provide research services for people with psychiatric disabilities. About 15 years ago, his focus broadened to the stigma of mental illness. He has had support from National Institute of Mental Health to develop and maintain the Chicago Consortium for Stigma Research (CCSR) for the past decade as its principal investigator. CCSR is a collection of more than a dozen researchers and advocates from academic and consumer groups in Northern Illinois. Dr Corrigan has authored more than 250 papers and 10 books. He is also the editor-in-chief for the *American Journal of Psychiatric Rehabilitation.*

Trevor P. Crowe, PhD, is a Research Fellow with the Illawarra Institute for Mental Health at the University of Wollongong. He currently coordinates a range of mental health and substance misuse clinician training and research programmes. Trevor is a Psychologist, Psychotherapist and Certified Addiction Counselor, with over 18 years of clinical experience. He has a particular interest in research and clinical work with people with comorbid mental health and substance misuse problems.

Frank P. Deane, PhD, is a Professor in the School of Psychology and Director of the Illawarra Institute for Mental Health at the University of Wollongong. He has worked in a range of clinical and academic positions in New Zealand, USA, and Australia. He teaches in the Clinical Psychology programmes and has research interests related to the effectiveness of mental health and substance abuse services, the role of therapeutic homework on treatment outcomes and help seeking for mental health and substance abuse problems.

Mandy W.M. Fong, BSc (Hons) in Psychology, is a Research Assistant at the Department of Rehabilitation Sciences, The Hong Kong Polytechnic University. She received her bachelor degree in psychology from the University of Nottingham, UK, in 2005. She is currently a master's student in the Department of Social Work and Social Administration at the University of

Hong Kong. Her research interests are on mental illness stigma, mental health promotion and rehabilitation.

Kelvin M.T. Fung, BSc (Hons), MPhil, is a doctoral candidate at the Department of Rehabilitation Sciences, The Hong Kong Polytechnic University. He received his bachelor degree in occupational therapy and master of philosophy in rehabilitation sciences in 2002 and 2006 respectively. His research interests have focused on mental illness stigma, mental health promotion and rehabilitation.

Robert King, PhD, is an Associate Professor in the School of Medicine (discipline of psychiatry) of the University of Queensland. He holds an MA (Clinical Psychology) from the University of Melbourne and a PhD from Monash University, and is a Fellow of the Australian Psychological Society and the College of Clinical Psychology. He publishes extensively in Australian and International peer-reviewed journals and has also made substantial contributions to published books. He is an Associate Editor for the US-based journal *Administration and Policy in Mental Health and Mental Health Services Research* and is the Peer Review Editor for *Psychotherapy in Australia*. In addition to research activities, he coordinates the University of Queensland's multidisciplinary mental health programme and is active in consultancy and staff training within and beyond Queensland.

Terry Krupa, PhD, is an Associate Professor in the School of Rehabilitation Therapy at Queen's University. She holds cross-appointments in the Department of Psychiatry and the School of Nursing, and is a Senior Adjunct Research Fellow with the University of South Australia. Her research and scholarly interests are in the area of disability, particularly related to mental illness, and includes work and productivity; activity and time use patterns and their relationship to well-being and citizenship; and service approaches that facilitate social and economic prosperity and full community inclusion.

Sally M.Y. Li, BSc (Hons) in Occupational Therapy, is a master of philosophy student at the Department of Rehabilitation Sciences, The Hong Kong Polytechnic University. She received her bachelor degree in occupational therapy in rehabilitation sciences from the Hong Kong Polytechnic University in 2002. Her research interests are on integrated supported employment, mental health promotion and rehabilitation.

Chris Lloyd, PhD, is a Senior Lecturer in the School of Population Health, The University of Queensland and the Queensland Centre for Mental Health Research. She received her undergraduate degree from the University of Alberta and her postgraduate degrees from the University of Queensland.

Dr Lloyd publishes extensively in peer-reviewed journals both in Australia and internationally, and has made substantial contributions to a number of published books. Her research and academic interests are in the areas of employment and people with a mental illness, leisure participation, family psychoeducation, and stress and burnout of mental health professionals.

Lindsay G. Oades, PhD, is a Senior Lecturer in the School of Psychology and the Illawarra Institute for Mental Health at the University of Wollongong. He teaches in the Clinical Psychology programmes and at the Sydney business school in Positive Psychology applications. His research focuses on the applications of positive psychological and goal striving applications in mental health recovery and health psychology.

Nikki Porteous, PG Cert (OT), Dip OT, NZROT, NZAOT, is an occupational therapist and the coordinator of WorkFirst and Individual Placement and Support (IPS) evidence-based supported employment service. WorkFirst is currently integrated with five Capital and Coast District Health Board community mental health teams in Wellington, New Zealand. She is a strong proponent of IPS and has co-published two articles with Dr Geoff Waghorn.

Christine E. Spowart, BScoSc, graduated from the University of Western Sydney with a Bachelor of Social Science (majoring in sociology and humanitarian and peace studies) in 2008. She has been in her current position as a Disability Employment Consultant, at a specialist mental health site, with break Thru People Solutions, since completing university. She is interested in combining her daily involvement with clients with research into best practice as well as trialling new strategies, with the purpose of empowering clients and improving their employment outcomes.

Hector W.H. Tsang, PhD, is the Associate Professor at the Department of Rehabilitation Sciences, The Hong Kong Polytechnic University. As an occupational therapist, he has an array of clinical experiences working with individuals with mental illness in hospital and community settings. As a researcher, his interests have focused on neuropsychiatric and vocational rehabilitation, mental illness stigma and psychophysiology of mind–body interventions. His research on social skills in the workplace won the Best Cross-regional Case Study Award in 1996 at the XIVth International Conference on the Social Sciences and Medicine organised by the International Forum for Social Sciences in Health (IFSSH), Scotland, UK. Dr Tsang has received a number of grants from various local and overseas funding bodies including the Public Policy Research Grant, Health and Health Services Research Grant, and Quality Education Fund in Hong Kong; and the

National Institute of Mental Health in the USA. In 2007, he spent his sabbatical at Yale University specialising his research on neurocognition and schizophrenia. He currently services on the editorial board of the *American Journal of Occupational Therapy*, the *American Journal of Psychiatric Rehabilitation*, and the *American Journal of Rehabilitation Counseling*. In addition, he is a reviewer of a number of prestigious journals including *Schizophrenia Bulletin*, *Schizophrenia Research*, *Psychiatry Research*, and the *Journal of Alternative and Complementary Medicine*.

Samson Tse, PhD, is currently Associate Professor at the Department of Social Work and Social Administration, The University of Hong Kong. His teaching and research focus is on recovery for individuals with psychiatric disability, in particular employment issues for people affected by bipolar disorder. Other research areas include problem gambling and cross-cultural health.

Niall Turner, BscOT, is the Occupational Therapy and Project Manager of the DETECT early intervention for psychosis service. He is also the Programmme Manager of the REACH Training Programme, a psychosocial rehabilitation programme which has been operational since 1995. He has worked in the rehabilitation field for over 10 years, in the last five focusing on occupational recovery in early psychosis. He has published research on psychosocial rehabilitation, employment and topics related to early intervention in psychosis. He is currently completing a masters by research with Trinity College Dublin. In 2009 he received funding to conduct a clinical trial of supported employment in an early intervention service from the Mental Health Commission in Ireland.

Geoff Waghorn, PhD, is a Principal Researcher for the Queensland Centre for Mental Health Research. Geoff holds a BSc (psychology major) from the University of Waitako, New Zealand, and post-graduate qualifications, including a PhD from the University of Queensland. He has an adjunct appointment as a Senior Lecturer in the School of Population Health, The University of Queensland. He leads a program of research into the functional recovery of people with mental illness and psychiatric disabilities. Current projects aim to reduce the social and economic marginalisation associated with mental illness and to improve the longer-term outcomes achieved by vocational and other non-treatment services. He has worked in the field of psychiatric disabilities in several roles, as a researcher for the past 10 years, previously as a clinical psychologist and rehabilitation consultant, and prior to that as a disability officer for a large Commonwealth Department. His current research interests are influenced by previous experiences in providing specialised psychiatric vocational rehabilitation services.

PREFACE

Employment in mental health services

Unemployment is harmful to health and is linked with increased general health problems. Unfortunately, unemployment can lead to social exclusion (Turner et al., 2009). It has been found that employment is beneficial in many aspects of people's lives, while not working can have detrimental effects on people's general health and well-being (Rinaldi et al., 2008). Work may be used to reintegrate people with mental illness into the community. As well as income, work provides other important benefits such as social identity and status, social contacts and support, a means of structuring and occupying time, activity and involvement, and a sense of personal achievement (Evans & Repper, 2000). The emphasis on social inclusion and integration rather than segregation has resulted in attempts to enable people with mental illness to gain and retain open employment through implementation of evidence-based practices in vocational services (Marwaha & Johnson, 2004).

Over the past several years, there has been very little change in the proportion of adults with mental illness participating in the workforce. This is in contrast with the increases of the employment rate in the general population and in those with physical disabilities. More concerning is the finding that the rates of employment for people with schizophrenia has actually decreased over the last decade (Perkins & Rinaldi, 2002). The lack of employment in those with severe mental illness, such as schizophrenia, is costly to society in terms of being in receipt of the disability allowance and not contributing to payment of taxes.

The increasing emphasis on productivity and the dominance of services industries and technology means that much of the nature of work has changed. This poses a problem for people with severe mental illness as they often have a poor work history and have problems with social skills (Tsang, 2001). These problems may be compounded by a lack of dedicated services helping people to obtain and to stay in work. There are also problems concerning being in receipt of disability allowances – the benefit trap – which may deter people from seeking employment. This may be particularly applicable for people considering working part-time. It seems that the main barriers to employment are stigmatisation of the mentally ill, economic disincentives, the attitudes and self-esteem of those with severe mental illness, and the response mental health services to their needs for support in obtaining and maintaining employment (Marwaha & Johnson, 2004). One of the biggest barriers to them finding and keeping work is that of stigma (Perkins et al., 2008).

It has been found that in most studies, the majority of respondents say they do want to work (McQuilken et al., 2003). However, it has been reported that people have concerns about receiving low pay and of being ashamed of their employment history and fears about their ability to cope with the work. These attitudes and beliefs can affect the likelihood of getting work and keeping it. Mental health professionals may unintentionally collude with barriers that people with mental illness face in gaining work. For example, vocational rehabilitation may not be included in the care plans of people with mental illness (Lehman & Steinwachs, 1998). The low expectations held by mental health professionals have been influenced by the dominance of a model for illness that emphasis symptoms and cure as opposed to a model of recovery. It may well be that mental health professionals may underestimate the skills, experiences and capabilities of their clients. These low expectations can create a cycle of decreasing hope and opportunity that has a direct impact on people with mental illness (Rinaldi et al., 2008).

There is an increasing interest in the subject of work for those with severe mental illness. This has arisen by the appearance of newer service models such as Individual Placement and Support (IPS; Bond et al., 2008). This model aims to assist clients get their chosen job and to provide the support they require to keep it rather than focusing exclusively on pre-vocational training. Potentially, this model has made employment for people with severe mental illness more achievable. It is thought that people with a mental illness are likely to regard meaningful recovery as involving a return to open market employment paid at a full usual rate. Seven core principles are included in this model. These principles include (1) a desire to work, (2) a focus on obtaining competitive employment, (3) an emphasis on rapid job placement, (4) the plan is individualised and based on consumer preference, (5) an integrated approach to service delivery, (6) follow-along supports are based on consumer needs rather than predetermined timeframes and (7) provision of benefits counselling.

This approach focuses on rapidly placing the person in a competitive employment situation, often within weeks after their initial enrolment in the programme (Corbiere & Lecomte, 2007). This is based on the client's choices and capabilities and does not require extended pre-vocational training. The employment specialist actively facilitates job acquisition. Staff tend to accompany clients on interviews, and they provide ongoing support once the client is employed. Most importantly, the IPS model integrates vocational and treatment teams. The major advantage of supported employment programmes over other vocational services is that the clients actually obtain real-world competitive jobs. This is important in promoting the client's role in society and facilitating their integration while working against the stigma of mental illness (Corbiere & Lecomte, 2007). But despite the increase in the number of programmes to assist people with severe mental illness find work, employment outcomes continue to be poor.

Various combinations, adaptations and integrations of specific vocational service components are used in order to help people with severe mental illness attain their vocational goals. It is important that practitioners become familiar with the types of approaches that have been developed, which augment vocational services. It is only be doing so that they will be better able to achieve more positive employment outcomes for their clients.

How the book is organised

Chapter 1 explores the impact that mental illness has on employment and looks at the value of work for people with mental illness.

Chapter 2 examines the evidence for supported employment services, in particular the IPS model.

Chapter 3 looks at the challenges of integrating mental health and employment services.

Chapter 4 examines the effect that stigma has on people with mental illness and looks at how supported employment may be used as an integrated employment strategy.

Chapter 5 looks at how motivational interviewing may be used as a means of assisting clients clarify and enhance motivation for change and resolve ambivalence about employment.

Chapter 6 examines the problems related for employment experienced by people with mental illness, in particular personal, environmental and occupational factors are addressed.

Chapter 7 examines the components thought to be important in the therapeutic relationship and in developing a strong therapeutic alliance in vocational rehabilitation contexts.

Chapter 8 suggests that a useful approach for practitioners to use is a recovery framework combining evidence-based employment and education assistance with mental health care provided in parallel with some other specific strategies.

Chapter 9 looks at the importance of planning and conducting employment programmes for young people with early psychosis.

Chapter 10 examines the importance of work-related social skills in job retention and outlines a protocol for integrated supported employment.

Chapter 11 looks at how symptoms of mental illness can interfere with employment outcomes and talks about various strategies to reduce the negative impact of symptoms.

Chapter 12 looks at the health benefits of education and describes the features and strategies that practitioners can employ to develop supported education programmes.

Chapter 13 talks about developing explicit plans with clients to comprehensively manage their personal information in order to access reasonable job accommodations.

Conclusions

Employment of people with mental illness has become an issue that has caught the attention of policy-makers. Researchers have demonstrated the effectiveness of the IPS approach to supported employment. It is now the time for mental health practitioners to consider the evidence for this approach to employment and look to using this information to better inform their practice. This book offers a variety of approaches and strategies designed to assist practitioners develop a comprehensive approach to assisting their clients find and maintain competitive employment.

References

Bond, G.R., Drake, R.E., & Becker, D.R. (2008). An update on randomized controlled trials of evidence-based supported employment. *Psychiatric Rehabilitation Journal, 31,* 280–290.

Corbiere, M., & Lecomte, T. (2007). Vocational services offered to people with severe mental illness. *Journal of Mental Health, 16,* 1–13.

Evans, J., & Repper, J. (2000). Employment, social inclusion and mental health. *Journal of Psychiatric and Mental Health Nursing, 7,* 15–24.

Lehman, A., & Steinwachs, D. (1998). Patterns of usual care for schizophrenia: initial results from the schizophrenia Patient Outcomes Research Team (PORT) client survey. *Schizophrenia Bulletin, 24,* 11–32.

Marwaha, S., & Johnson, S. (2004). Schizophrenia and employment: a review. *Social Psychiatry and Psychiatric Epidemiology, 39,* 337–349.

McQuilken, M., Zahniser, J.H., Novak, J., Starks, R.D., Olmos, A., & Bond, G.R. (2003). The work project survey: consumer perspectives on work. *Journal of Vocational Rehabilitation, 18,* 59–68.

Perkins, D.V., Rainer, J.A., Tschopp, M.K., & Warner, T.C. (2008). Gainful employment reduces stigma toward people recovering from schizophrenia. *Community Mental Health Journal, 45,* 158–162.

Perkins, R., & Rinaldi, M. (2002). Unemployment rates among patients with long term mental health problems. *Psychiatric Bulletin, 26,* 295–298.

Rinaldi, M., Perkins, R., Glynn, E., Montibeller, T., Clenaghan, M., & Rutherford, J. (2008). Individual placement and support: from research to practice. *Advances in Psychiatric Treatment, 13,* 50–60.

Tsang, H.W.H. (2001). Applying social skills training in the context of vocational rehabilitation for people with schizophrenia. *The Journal of Nervous and Mental Disease, 189,* 90–98.

Turner, N., Browne, S., Clarke, M., Gervin, M., Larkin, C., Waddington, J.L., & O'Callaghan, E. (2009). Employment status amongst those with psychosis at first presentation. *Social Psychiatry and Psychiatric Epidemiology, 44,* 863–869.

Chapter 1

EMPLOYMENT AND PEOPLE WITH MENTAL ILLNESS

Geoff Waghorn and Chris Lloyd

Chapter overview

This chapter explores the impact of mental illness on employment. It goes on to talk about the value of employment and how people with a mental illness have both the capacity and the desire to work. There are a number of barriers to employment, ranging from the nature of the disorder, stigma and career immaturity. Today, recovery is an important concept and we talk about how employment and education contribute to recovery. We conclude the chapter by examining evidence-based interventions that will assist people in achieving their goal of competitive employment.

Introduction

There is substantial evidence that the vocational rehabilitation needs of people with mental illness are not being adequately addressed. Labour force non-participation and unemployment levels of 75–90% are found in the USA (Hughes, 1999), 61–73% in the UK, and reach 75–78% among people with psychotic disorders in Australia (Waghorn et al., 2004a). In countries with developed market economies, people with mental illness experience difficulties in achieving the basic right to work (Harnois & Gabriel, 2000). They are also sensitive to the negative effects of unemployment and the loss of purpose, structure, roles, status and sense of identity, which employment provides (Boardman et al., 2003). Employment enables social inclusion in the wider community and represents an important way in which people with mental illness can meaningfully participate in society. People with mental illness need the same opportunities to participate in life activities and their local communities as people with good mental health (Corrigan, 2003). All people in our community have the right to suitable employment in conditions which reflect equity, security, human dignity and respect. Work is important to the mental health and wellbeing of individuals. It is a central aspect of life for most people and provides economic security, valued personal roles, social identity and an opportunity to make a meaningful contribution to the community. Suitable employment enables social and economic participation in society.

This chapter aims to discuss how mental illness can cause barriers to employment and identify the evidence-based ingredients to employment assistance.

The impact of mental illness on employment

Anxiety and depression are prevalent in the community and together are found in approximately 5–10% of the population (Australian Bureau of Statistics, 1998) at any time. Anxiety disorders are associated with increased non-participation in the labour force, deflated employment trajectories and impaired work performance compared to healthy people (Waghorn et al., 2005b).

Depression is known to cause absenteeism from work (Kessler & Frank, 1997) and impair work performance when at work (Kessler et al., 2001). People with depression also have reduced labour force participation, reduced working hours and may earn less than healthy workers (Whooley et al., 2002). People with depression may have impaired motivation, impaired decision-making and a reduced capacity to initiate a particular course of action. Depression can be misunderstood by employers and vocational service providers as poor motivation for work generally or, when employed, as low motivation for working productively.

Bipolar disorder can fluctuate more than most other mental disorders, and may involve a manic phase where productivity and creativity can be high, time and energy management may be impaired and the person may over-exert themselves until a depression cycle is reached. People with bipolar affective disorders may have relatively little difficulty obtaining employment, but unless new strategies are learned to monitor warning signs (e.g. increasing energy, productivity and creativity at work; or increasing social withdrawal at work and difficulty getting to work) job retention is likely to be the major issue.

The onset of mental illness can permanently disrupt education, employment and career development (Waghorn et al., 2004b). Although of low point prevalence compared to anxiety and depression at approximately 0.47% of the population, mental illness is associated with a lifelong career disruption. Despite evidence of career disruption, long-term outcome studies (Harding et al., 1987) and successful vocational programmes (Bond et al., 1995) support the feasibility of employment for a substantial proportion of persons with mental illness.

Employment restrictions among people with mental illness

At a population level the most commonly reported employment restrictions among people with anxiety disorders are restricted in the type of job (24.0%), need for a support person (23.3%), difficulty in changing jobs (18.6%) and restricted in the number of hours (15.4%). A substantial proportion of people with anxiety disorders (23.3%) and 61.3% of people with psychotic disorders (Waghorn & Chant, 2005) report a need for a support person if participating in employment. The psychotic disorders are associated with the greatest proportions of employment restrictions. However, substantial proportions of people with depression and anxiety disorders also report employment restrictions.

The impact of mental illness on education and vocational training

The onset of mental illness can truncate primary, secondary or tertiary educational attainment and vocational training, and disrupt normal career development. For psychotic disorders, this may occur because the typical onset age is from 10 to 30 years, which may coincide with the critical career stages of completing formal education and establishing a career pathway. Through disrupting education, mental illness can indirectly cause long-term unemployment and limit career prospects. Hence, mental illness can displace career paths downwards and limit attainment to less skilled jobs, lowering both work status and income expectations.

Several studies have identified the importance of education to career development. A longitudinal study (Mueser et al., 2001a) and a secondary analysis of data (Mechanic et al., 2002) linked educational attainment to increased employment outcomes and higher employment status in the USA. In Australia, educational attainment is closely associated with employment outcomes. Waghorn et al. (2002) found positive links between educational attainment and both current employment and durable employment among people with psychotic disorders.

The need for specialised treatments to reduce employment restrictions

People with mental disorders can have difficulty obtaining both optimal treatment and suitable vocational assistance. They may be turned away by practitioners who recognise the extensive employment restrictions associated with the severe forms of these disorders. Practitioners may be unwilling or unable to provide specialist psychological and psychiatric treatments as part of a comprehensive vocational rehabilitation plan. However, specialised psychological treatments coordinated by a vocational plan may be particularly effective through leveraging treatment motivation with vocational motivation. Providing timely and effective supplementary treatment is, therefore, likely to reduce employment restrictions and increase the prospect of favourable vocational outcomes. Specialised treatment need not delay vocational plans because these can be provided in parallel with vocational interventions.

Capacity and desire for work

Non-participation in the labour force and high unemployment do not mean that people with mental illness are incapable of working. Studies of the long-term course of illness and health outcomes of people with schizophrenia (Mechanic et al., 2002) have found substantial heterogeneity of course and outcome, with improvement over time in social functioning in 40–70% of people previously classified as having the most severe disabilities. Controlled studies of the effectiveness of supported employment (Bond et al., 2004) demonstrate the feasibility of competitive employment, even when no screening criteria other than the initial interest determine programme entry. Bond et al. (2004) found that 40–60% of consumers receiving evidence-based supported employment assistance obtained competitive employment. Long-term outcome research and controlled studies of supported employment support the feasibility of psychiatric vocational rehabilitation for people with mental illness, including a substantial proportion of persons with the most severe forms of schizophrenia.

Labour force non-participation and high unemployment do not imply that people with mental illness do not want to work. Low labour force participation may represent discouraged job seeking or loss of vocational hope, because a substantial proportion of mental health service consumers with severe mental illness consider employment feasible and a key element to their recovery (Liberman et al., 2002). When specifically prompted, consumers frequently state that they want employment (Davidson & McGlashan, 1997) even when mental health providers rate employment as a low priority (Fischer et al., 2002). Other qualitative studies (Honey, 2000) have found that people with a severe mental illness actively strive to obtain meaningful roles and an appropriate vocational place in the community.

Value of employment

Rowland and Perkins (1988) identified four benefits of work: work as a restorative psychological process, work to improve self-concept, the protective effect of work and the social dimension of work. Positive and meaningful employment experiences have been linked to improved self-concept and self-efficacy (Strong, 1998), higher ratings of subjective well-being (Laird & Krown, 1991), regaining self-esteem (Van Dongen, 1996), improved engagement in work activity with associated symptom reduction (Bell et al., 1996) and increased personal empowerment (Rogers et al., 1997). Work may also improve clinical insight for those with severe mental illness who have less severe cognitive impairments (Lysaker et al., 1995).

Reviews of randomised controlled trials (Bond et al., 2004) reveal that the main benefit of supported employment is on short-term individual employment outcomes. Other benefits associated with work include structuring time and routine, social contact, collective effort and purpose, social identity and status, personal achievement, and regular activity and involvement (Boardman et al., 2003).

However, job retention challenges all forms of employment assistance (Xie et al., 1997), indicating that continuing support to retain employment is critical for people with mental illness. Although there is evidence that sustained employment enhances the non-vocational outcomes of improved self-esteem and symptom control, there is no consistent evidence that employment leads to reduced hospitalisations or improves quality of life (Bond et al., 2001a, b). Despite these evidence gaps, suitable and meaningful employment can be highly valued by individuals. The following account (S.T Scott, personal communication to MIFA, March 2005) illustrates the personal value of employment:

> *'I have found that working part-time has definitely given me the positive edge on a more healthy self-esteem. Working has taken away the dread of socialising and meeting new people as to when I am asked in conversation, what I do for a living. Once upon a time I had the embarrassment of saying nothing or else saying that I was on a disability pension. Then there was the fear that they would inquire more deeply and I would be exposed as explaining I had a mental illness. With a large portion of society ignorant about mental illness and still having stigma, this position would further squash an already low self-esteem. Working has given me the opportunity to flee this scenario as well as giving me structure and routine.*
>
> *If I have days or weeks where I'm starting to get slightly unwell, work is the best therapy for me. It gets my eyes off myself and focussed on to others' needs. Being employed as a supervisor of an Activity Drop-In centre for people with a mental illness, I find serving others needs and healing is good for the soul. I have discovered that the best way to help yourself is simply by helping someone else. With mental health issues, loneliness and boredom are a good recipe for becoming unwell and work has structured my time, so even if I feel lazy and unmotivated, I have to get into action and attend and perform in my job. For people who are ready to take the next step of some degree of work I encourage the system to give them every opportunity as it is vital to that road to recovery.'*

Reducing workplace and community stigma

People with mental illness experience considerable stigma and discrimination (Waghorn & Lewis, 2002) from both employers and the general community. Practitioners can counter the stigma associated with mental illness by strategic disclosure to employers and to other third parties throughout vocational rehabilitation. They have the opportunity to counter community stigma by enabling people with mental illness to demonstrate their work potential. Personal contact with people experiencing mental illness in the workplace, supported by planned education of managers, supervisors and co-workers, may counter stigma both in the workplace and in the wider community.

How mental illness produces barriers to employment

Employment barriers can result from the positive, negative and disorganised symptoms of psychosis, from side effects of antipsychotic, mood stabilising and antidepressant medications, and from subsequent impairments to social skills, sense of self, personal confidence and self-efficacy (Anthony, 1994). In addition, indirect barriers to employment can result from the negative experiences of stigma and unfair discrimination, and from the timing of illness onset which can disrupt formal education and training, impede school-to-work transitions and damage the formation of work values and core work skills.

Cognitive impairments

Mental illness can produce cognitive, perceptual, affective and interpersonal deficits, each of which may contribute to employment barriers (Rutman, 1994). Of these, the cognitive deficits have a more consistent association with unemployment (Tsang et al., 2000) and poor work performance. Cognitive deficits consistently found in schizophrenia or schizoaffective disorder includes generalised deficits such as lowered full-scale IQ and a reduced capacity for information processing (Lewis, 2004). Specific deficits can include problems with attention, sustained attention, memory and executive functioning (Lewis, 2004).

Cognitive symptoms are likely to cause employment restrictions which limit occupational choice through restricting the type of work activities which can be successfully performed. Industry and job choices can be restricted, work hours and work performance may be limited, and the need for ongoing assistance to retain employment may be increased (McGurk et al., 2003). In addition, general cognitive deficits as well as deficits in social cognition are associated with impaired work-related social skills, and may underlie the impaired social competence which can influence vocational outcomes (Tsang et al., 2000).

Other clinical symptoms

Almost all the clinical symptoms associated with mental illness can, at an individual level, directly contribute to employment barriers. Clinical symptoms may impair social skills development. Psychiatric symptoms are potentially disabling and can vary over time, yet are not consistent predictors of vocational outcomes. Tsang et al. (2000) reviewed controlled studies between 1985 and 1997 and found in particular that diagnostic category and psychiatric symptoms were inconsistent predictors. The most consistent predictors of employment outcomes were found to be work history, premorbid functioning and current social skills.

The episodic nature of the disorders

Mental illnesses can be episodic and fluctuating in nature despite optimal pharmacological treatment and good psychological and social support. The first and subsequent episodes can be frightening and traumatic experiences which damage a person's stability and identity, thus weakening their ability to commit to longer term endeavours such as vocational rehabilitation (Rutman, 1994). In addition, during relatively stable periods people can have their assistance needs underestimated by providers of housing, disability, income, family and employment assistance, which can lead to refusal of services or under-provision of support, leading to adverse events causing frustration and hopelessness, further weakening the person's capacity to manage vocational challenges. A way to assess career-related assistance needs is to take account of predictors and correlates of employment outcomes, namely level of employment restrictions, lifelong pattern of illness, premorbid functioning, educational attainment, relevant work history, relevant vocational skills and current social skills (Waghorn et al., 2005a).

Treatment interventions as indirect barriers to employment

Both pharmacological and psychological treatment interventions can produce additional barriers to obtaining and retaining employment. The known side effects of anti-psychotic, antidepressant and mood stabilising medications and the time taken to establish optimal medication type and dosage can cause difficulties for the provision of vocational assistance. In addition, suboptimal treatment can contribute to poor adherence, which in turn can exacerbate symptoms, interfere with planned treatment and undermine vocational interventions.

Treatment and vocational rehabilitation interventions need to be coordinated so that changes to treatment plans (e.g. a new medication trial) do not conflict with planned vocational activities. Sometimes treatment goals need to be balanced by vocational goals. For instance, some residual positive symptoms may be preferred to a symptom-free state with lowered energy levels, insufficient to sustain preferred hours of employment. Failure to actively coordinate interventions may create a barrier to employment, placing the onus on the person least likely to manage this responsibility.

Low vocational expectations by health professionals

Blankertz and Robinson (1996) believe that health professionals' low vocational expectations of service users is a major problem because it prevents the majority of people from receiving vocational rehabilitation and supported employment services. Mental health professionals often report that people with mental illness have unrealistic work expectations and goals (Becker et al., 1998). In examining programmes with low rates of people with mental illness in competitive employment, it was found that the onus was left on individuals to bring up their interests in employment with the service provider. In addition, service providers tended to emphasise prevocational programmes devoted to job preparation, did not pursue rapid assessment to capitalise on the service users' motivation for work, had limited contact with vocational services, had little direct employer contact and provided minimal support to people once they were in employment (Gowdy et al., 2003).

Community stigma

In general, the public does not understand the impact of mental illness and frequently fears people with these disorders. Members of the community withhold opportunities related to housing, work and community participation (Corrigan, 2003). People with mental illness have fewer opportunities to work than the general population, mostly owing to the many misperceptions and prejudices about their abilities and needs. They are not expected to work, and indeed they are often considered not fit or well enough to work (Evans & Repper, 2000). The lack of work serves to reinforce negative stereotypes and social exclusion associated with mental illness. By not appearing within employment settings, it is mistakenly believed that people with mental illness are too incapacitated to work (Evans & Repper, 2000). An additional issue is that some people with mental illness also endorse stigmatising attitudes about mental illness. This internalised stigma affects the individual's self-perception and has the potential to impact on the success or failure of employment opportunities (Caltruax, 2003).

Community stigma and unfair discrimination are frequently reported by people with mental illness (World Health Organisation, 2001) as adding to the difficulties of obtaining and retaining employment. The extent of past stigma experiences and reactions to those experiences can influence personal decisions about whether or not vocational goals are adopted. In addition, past stigma experiences may exert a strong influence on disclosure preferences throughout psychiatric vocational rehabilitation (Waghorn & Lewis, 2002). To overcome the adverse effects of prior community stigma, vocational professionals can provide stigma assessment and counselling and develop ongoing stigma countering and disclosure strategies within every individual's vocational rehabilitation plan.

Workplace stigma

The attitudes of employers towards people with mental illness may reflect the ignorance and stigma prevalent in the wider community (Waghorn & Lewis, 2002). This then may result in the belief that people with mental illness are unable to work or that it is not possible to accommodate psychiatric disorders within the workplace. Negative employer attitudes have a number of implications, including that an employer will not hire a person with psychiatric disability or advance or retain people with these disorders (Spillane, 1999). When a person with a mental illness is hired, they may be treated differently from other workers. For example, Murphy (1998) reported that people with mental illness faced discrimination and prejudice by employers and co-workers once they knew the person had a disability. This included that the employer began to be afraid of the person, verbal abuse, harassment and belittling the person's ability and judgement.

Career immaturity

Mental illness can create unique individual experiences, which can lead to inappropriate values, attitudes and aspirations regarding work and careers (Rutman, 1994). Impaired work values and impaired perceptions of current work skills can cause unrealistic vocational goals, where perceptions of own work skills may diverge from actual skill levels and experience. These experiences may also represent career immaturity thought to result from the lack of exposure to typical life experiences, responsibilities and roles which help a person form appropriate work perceptions, work confidence, work interests, work values and work ethics. Although the precise psychological processes are unclear, it is likely that career maturity is influenced by the person's life experiences, personality, perceptions of illness experiences, family background, educational attainment, work values, and knowledge of workplaces and employer requirements.

Subjective experiences and personal resources

Internal barriers to achieving vocational goals include unpredictable sleeping patterns, fear of failure, fear of relapse, lack of confidence in vocational abilities, difficulties with concentration and fear of resuming work after years of unemployment (Corrigan, 2003). In addition, Waghorn et al. (2005a) found that a range of varied subjective experiences perceived to impact on work functioning and self-efficacy for specific work-related activities were closely associated with employment status.

Mallick et al. (1998) found that financial resources, employment resources and vocational skills presented the greatest barriers to community integration. Financial resources included money for meeting financial obligations such as rent, food and other daily expenses. Employment resources were employment opportunities and available resources to find a job and maintain employment. Waghorn et al. (2005a) found that self-efficacy for core employment activities includes career planning, job-securing skills, job-retaining work skills (e.g. start work soon after arriving, complete tasks in the time required, identify and correct own mistakes) and job-retaining social skills (e.g. can follow instructions without resistance, can cooperate with co-workers to perform a group task, can check instructions with supervisors).

Vocational interventions and a recovery framework

Recovery is defined as the process of overcoming symptoms, psychiatric disability and social handicap. It can involve a redefinition of the self, the emergence of hope and optimism, empowerment and the establishment of meaningful relationships with others (Resnick et al., 2004). Recovery is oriented towards the reconstruction of meaning and purpose in one's life, the performance of valued social roles, the experience of mental health and well-being and life satisfaction. It means maximising well-being within the constraints imposed by health status. A recovery framework incorporates continuing care with relapse prevention plans and psychosocial rehabilitation (see Chapter 8 for a detailed discussion on the importance of vocation in recovery). The lived experience of the person with the mental illness is also acknowledged and attempts are made to maximise their well-being along with that of their family (Rickwood, 2004).

As an evidence-based form of psychosocial rehabilitation, vocational rehabilitation is ideally suited to a recovery framework. Recovery planning can incorporate a discussion of preferred socially valued roles, and if vocational roles are chosen, vocational activities can become the focus of the recovery plan. A comprehensive recovery plan can also include crisis planning, a list of things that people have done in the past to help themselves to stay well and a list of things they could do to help themselves feel better when things are not going well (Rickwood, 2004).

How employment and education contribute to recovery

Work has an important role in the recovery of people with mental illness and many of the goals of rehabilitation are best served by addressing the person's vocational aspirations (Corrigan, 2003). Employment contributes to the recovery process through being perceived as a means of self-empowerment and by promoting a sense of self-actualisation (Provencher et al., 2002). Meaningful activities can also contribute to the recovery process through active participation in structured social, recreational, volunteer work, arts and education.

Evidence-based vocational interventions

Various vocational interventions suitable for people with mental illness have evolved over time. Although each approach to vocational assistance has its advocates, a positive development in the literature is a new focus on the ingredients of effective vocational rehabilitation specifically designed for people with mental illness. Vocational interventions for people with mental illness have included unpaid voluntary work, the Boston University psychiatric rehabilitation model (Choose-Get-Keep) with extended pre-vocational career exploration, job clubs (Corrigan et al., 1995), the Programme of Assertive Community Treatment, generic supported employment, Clubhouse transitional employment, specialised supported employment (also known as the Individual Placement and Support model of supported employment), generic vocational rehabilitation and specialised vocational rehabilitation (Waghorn & King, 1999).

In addition, there are interventions such as business services (sheltered workshops), work crews, community cooperatives and social firms. These services are usually designed to increase employment opportunities for people with disabilities by providing supportive and low stigma work environments and by producing goods or services in order to pursue employment as a social justice mission. In social firms, the proportion of disadvantaged workers does not exceed 30–50% and every worker is paid an industrial award wage or a productivity-based wage. Both disabled and healthy workers are intended to have equality in terms of opportunities, rights and responsibilities.

Unique principles of transitional employment

Although on-site support is commonly provided in supported employment and vocational rehabilitation, an important and unique principle of Clubhouse transitional employment programmes is the continuous availability of intensive on-site support (Bilby, 1999). This aims to overcome employment barriers in the workplace by demonstrating core work skills and appropriate work behaviours, using on-site training to teach and reinforce good work attitudes, behaviours and performance. Consequently, the close relationship formed between Clubhouse staff and employers enables a suitable training environment to be created for assisting new members at work and for countering stigma by educating others in the workplace about mental illness and mental health.

Transitional employment is a form of psychiatric vocational rehabilitation developed specifically for people with psychiatric disabilities (Henry et al., 2000). Intensive forms of on-site assistance are routinely provided at each entry-level job held by the Clubhouse. Staff members learn the job in order to perform the duties on days when the member(s) selected to perform the job for a specified period is unwell or unable to attend. The aim is to provide members with real employment experiences (paid-at-award wages) to overcome career immaturity and to help people form and test career goals. Transitional employment placements are typically part-time, linked to prior participation in Clubhouse day programmes (the work-ordered day) and limited to a duration of 4–6 months, to enable other members to share the available opportunities. Clubhouses may also offer housing, social recreation and supported education programmes.

Although not formally identified as contributing to employment outcomes, the Clubhouse member-based organisation provides an appropriate infrastructure for people with mental illness. Like social firms, Clubhouses provide safe low-stigma environments which encourage vocational recovery and support general illness recovery through peer support, sharing of resources and increased social and recreational opportunities to help rebuild personal and social confidence.

Principles of specialised supported employment

Specialised supported employment (Drake et al., 2003) is important for both its evidence base of randomised controlled trials and day-centre conversion projects and for the empirical identification of its underlying theoretical principles. Previously known as the Individual Placement and Support (IPS) approach to supported employment, evidence is accumulating that this form of specialised supported employment is effective for 40–60% of volunteers (Lucca et al., 2004). A consensus is emerging as to the evidence-base for each of the seven principles while research efforts continue to identify programme enhancements. According to Bond (2004), there is consistent evidence for the first four of the following seven principles, while the evidence for the latter three remain relatively weak:

(1) Eligibility based on consumer choice
(2) Integration of vocational rehabilitation with mental health care

(3) A goal of competitive employment
(4) Rapid commencement of job search activities
(5) Services based on consumer preferences
(6) Continuing support to retain employment
(7) Income support and health benefits counselling.

Service eligibility is based on consumer choice (Bond et al., 2001c). No attempt is made to screen out participants on grounds other than individual preferences and motivation. This approach has been found to be more effective when integrated within the mental health treatment team (Mueser et al., 2004). Integration is considered advantageous in four ways: (1) better engagement and retention of clients, (2) better communication between employment specialists and clinicians, (3) education of clinicians about employment issues and (4) incorporation of clinical information into vocational plans (Drake et al., 2003).

The main goal is competitive employment rather than participation in day programmes or sheltered work, which are usually not provided. The evidence suggests that interventions not focusing directly on competitive employment have little or no impact on competitive employment outcomes (Bond, 2004). In addition, competitive employment outcomes are more desirable and recovery oriented than other forms of paid employment. The early use of supported job searching and job placement is considered important to prevent people from losing interest in the necessary elements of job preparation and training in specific job skills.

Other interventions when provided are done so in parallel and not in series with job searching or job placement. Bell et al. (2003) found that cognitive skills training provided concurrently with supported employment was a successful parallel intervention which need not delay either job searching or job placement. Both treatment and vocational interventions are tailored to the type of job searching or work tasks required.

Services provided are based on consumer preferences, strengths, prior work interests and experiences rather than on a pool of available jobs. The evidence shows that the majority of clients have stable and realistic job preferences (Becker et al., 1998) and jobs matched to the initial job preference had a longer job tenure than those not so matched (Mueser et al., 2001b).

Follow-on support is available continuously over time with no closure date, so that on-the-job or behind-the-scenes support is available when needed. Employment specialists stay in regular contact with clients and employers without arbitrary time limits, although the intensity of support may reduce to a maintenance level of regular contact only. McHugo et al. (1998) found supporting evidence at 3.5 years from the commencement of employment, where 71% of those who continued receiving support were still employed, compared to 28% of those who had discontinued support. Support is provided proactively and in partnership with the person with mental illness.

Health and welfare benefits counselling is provided, although the current supporting evidence is relatively weak (Bond, 2004). Consumers are helped to make well-informed decisions about their entitlements to welfare benefits and health insurance coverage to ensure that benefits entitlements do not add unnecessary disincentives to employment.

Emerging candidates for evidence-based components

The use of explicit strategies to counter workplace stigma and structured counselling to optimise disclosure strategies are also expected to enhance outcomes in psychiatric vocational rehabilitation by improving job commencement and job retention. Some people may fail to seek, obtain or retain employment because of past stigma experiences or previous workplace discrimination (Spillane, 1999). Hence, strategies are needed throughout vocational rehabilitation to counter past and present stigma and strategically manage disclosure of personal mental health information in the workplace (Waghorn & Lewis, 2002).

To prevent negative stigma experiences in a particular workplace, a plan for workplace education can be developed along with the vocational rehabilitation plan. Initial education can be provided to increase mental health literacy generally and to counter stigma-based beliefs prevalent at the supervisory and managerial level (Spillane, 1999). Mental illnesses such as anxiety disorders, depression and even schizophrenia can be discussed in the context of occupational health and safety, the work environment, and general mental health and well-being, which are topics of interest in most workplaces. Ongoing support plans for the individual can encompass a plan to increase mental health literacy, and to prevent and counter stigma in the workplace over time. This can be achieved by (1) facilitating co-worker social interaction, (2) teaching specific work-related social skills to the worker with the mental illness, (3) using peer support arrangements, (4) ongoing strategic and ethical disclosure of health information relevant to work performance and (5) planned ongoing education of employers, supervisors, co-workers and third parties throughout the vocational rehabilitation process.

However, some people may report such negative stigma experiences that they are currently unwilling to consider an open employment placement. For these people, stigma-safe environments may be needed to enable rebuilding of work and social confidence. Hence, to meet a broad spectrum of assistance needs, alternatives to open employment approaches, such as transitional employment, business services, social firms and community cooperatives, can contribute by providing low-stigma work environments as a bridging option towards open employment.

Conclusions

This chapter has reviewed the impact of mental illness on employment. Employment has many advantages for people. People with a mental illness have the capacity and the desire for work; however, their employment is impeded by a number of factors. Practitioners becoming aware and adopting the evidence-based vocational interventions is a key step in assisting people to participate in a socially valued role. Vocational interventions need to focus on eligibility based on consumer choice, integration of vocational rehabilitation in mental health employment, a goal of competitive employment and rapid commencement of job search activities.

References

Anthony, W.A. (1994). Characteristics of people with psychiatric disabilities that are predictive of entry into the rehabilitation process and successful employment. *Psychosocial Rehabilitation Journal, 17*, 3–13.

Australian Bureau of Statistics. (1998). *Mental Health and Wellbeing: Profile of Adults.* Cat no. 4326.0. Canberra, Australia: Commonwealth Government, Australian Bureau of Statistics.

Becker, D.R., Bebout, R.R., & Drake, R.E. (1998). Job preferences of people with severe mental illness: a replication. *Psychiatric Rehabilitation Journal, 22*, 46–50.

Bell, M., Lysaker, P., & Bryson, G. (2003). A behavioural intervention to improve work performance in schizophrenia: work behaviour inventory feedback. *Journal of Vocational Rehabilitation, 18*, 43–50.

Bell, M.D., Lysaker, P.H., & Milstein, R.M. (1996). Clinical benefits of paid work activity in schizophrenia. *Schizophrenia Bulletin, 22*, 51–67.

Bilby, R. (1999). Transitional employment: the most supported of supported employments. *The Clubhouse Community Journal, 1*, 34–36.

Blankertz, R., & Robinson, S. (1996). Adding a vocational focus to mental health rehabilitation. *Psychiatric Services, 47*, 1216–1222.

Boardman, J., Grove, B., Perkins, R., & Shepherd, G. (2003). Work and employment for people with psychiatric disabilities. *British Journal of Psychiatry, 182*, 467–468.

Bond, G. (2004). Supported Employment: evidence for an evidence-based practice. *Psychiatric Rehabilitation Journal, 27*, 345–359.

Bond, G., Resnick, S.R., Drake, R.E., Xie, H., McHugo, G.J., & Bebout, R.R. (2001b). Does competitive employment improve non-vocational outcomes for people with severe mental illness? *Journal of Consulting and Clinical Psychology, 69*, 489–501.

Bond, G., Salyers, M., Rollins, A., Rapp, C., & Zipple, A. (2004). How evidence-based practices contribute to community integration. *Community Mental Health Journal, 40*, 569–588.

Bond, G.R., Becker, D.R., Drake, R.E., Rapp, C.A., Meisler, N., Lehman, A.F., Bell, M.D., & Blyler, C.R. (2001a). Implementing supported employment as an evidenced based practice. *Psychiatric Services, 52*, 313–322.

Bond, G.R., Becker, D.R., Drake, R.E., Rapp, C.A., Meisler, N., Lehman, A.F., Bell, M.D., & Blyler, C.R. (2001c). Implementing supported employment as an evidenced based practice. *Psychiatric Services, 52*, 313–322.

Bond, G.R., Dietzen, L.L., McGrew, J.H., & Miller, L.D. (1995). Accelerated entry into supported employment for persons with severe psychiatric disabilities. *Rehabilitation Psychology, 40*, 75–94.

Caltruax, D. (2003). Internalized stigma: a barrier to employment for people with mental illness. *International Journal of Therapy and Rehabilitation, 10*, 539–543.

Corrigan, P., Reedy, P., Thadani, D., & Ganet, M. (1995). Correlates of participation and completion in a job club for clients with psychiatric disability. *Rehabilitation Counseling Bulletin, 39*, 43–53.

Corrigan, P.W. (2003). Beat the stigma: come out of the closet. *Psychiatric Services, 54*, 1313.

Davidson, L., & McGlashan, T.H. (1997). The varied outcomes of schizophrenia. *Canadian Journal of Psychiatry, 42*, 34–43.

Drake, R.E., Becker, D.R., Bond, G.R., & Mueser, K.T. (2003). A process analysis of integrated and non-integrated approaches to supported employment. *Journal of Vocational Rehabilitation, 18*, 51–58.

Evans, J., & Repper, J. (2000). Employment, social inclusion and mental health. *Journal of Psychiatric and Mental Health Nursing, 7*, 15–24.

Fischer, E.P., Shumway, M., & Owen, R.R. (2002). Priorities of consumers, providers and family members in the treatment of schizophrenia. *Psychiatric Services, 53*, 724–729.

Gowdy, E.A., Carlson, L.S., & Rapp, C.A. (2003). Practices differentiating high-performing from low-performing supported employment programs. *Psychiatric Rehabilitation Journal, 26*, 232–239.

Harding, C.M., Brooks, G.W., Ashikaga, T., Strauss, J.S., & Breier, A. (1987). The Vermont longitudinal study of persons with severe mental illness. II: Long-term outcome of subjects who retrospectively met DSM-III criteria for schizophrenia. *American Journal of Psychiatry, 144*, 727–735.

Harnois, G., & Gabriel, P. (2000). *Mental Health and Work: Impact, Issues and Good Practices*. Geneva: World Health Organization and International Labour Organisation.

Henry, A.D., Barreira, P., Banks, S., Brown, J., & McKay, C. (2000). A retrospective study of clubhouse based transitional employment. *Psychiatric Rehabilitation Journal, 24*, 344–354.

Honey, A. (2000). Psychiatric vocational rehabilitation: where are the customers' views? *Psychiatric Rehabilitation Journal, 23*, 270–279.

Hughes, R. (1999). Psychosocial rehabilitation: new protocols, ethics and outcomes. *International Journal of Mental Health, 28*, 3–33.

Kessler R., & Frank R. (1997). The impact of psychiatric disorders on work loss days. *Psychological Medicine, 27*, 861–873.

Kessler, R.C., Greenberg, P.E., Mickelson, K.D., Meneades, L.M., & Wang, P.S. (2001). The effects of chronic medical conditions on work loss and work cutback. *Journal of Occupational & Environmental Medicine, 43*, 218–225.

Laird, M., & Krown, S. (1991). Evaluation of a transitional employment program. *Psychosocial Rehabilitation Journal, 15*, 3–8.

Lewis, R. (2004). Should cognitive deficit be a diagnostic criterion for schizophrenia? *Journal of Psychiatry Neuroscience, 29*, 102–113.

Liberman, R.P., Kopelowicz, A., Ventura, J., & Gutkind, D. (2002). Operational criteria and factors related to recovery from schizophrenia. *International Review of Psychiatry*, *14*, 256–272.

Lucca, A.M., Henry, A.D., Banks, S., Simon, L., & Page, S. (2004). Evaluation of an Individual Placement and Support model program. *Psychiatric Rehabilitation Journal*, *27*, 251–257.

Lysaker, P.H., Bell, M.D., & Bioty, M.S. (1995). Cognitive deficits in schizophrenia: prediction of symptom change for participants in work rehabilitation. *Journal of Nervous and Mental Disease*, *183*, 332–336.

Mallick, K., Reeves, R., & Dellario, D. (1998). Barriers to community integration for people with severe and persistent disabilities. *Psychiatric Rehabilitation Journal*, *22*, 175–180.

McGurk, S.R., Mueser, K.T., Harvey, P.D., La Puglia, R., & Marder, J. (2003). Cognitive and symptom predictors of work outcomes for clients with schizophrenia in supported employment. *Psychiatric Services*, *54*, 1129–1135.

McHugo, G.J., Drake, R.E., & Becker, D.R. (1998). The durability of supported employment effects. *Psychiatric Rehabilitation Journal*, *22*, 55–61.

Mechanic, D., Bilder, S., & McAlpine, D.D. (2002). Employment of persons with serious mental illness. *Health Affairs*, *21*, 242–249.

Mueser, K.T., Becker, D.R., & Wolfe, R.S. (2001b). Supported employment, job preferences, job tenure and satisfaction. *Journal of Mental Health*, *10*, 411–417.

Mueser, K.T., Clark, R.E., Haines, M., Drake, R.E., McHugo, G, J., Bond, G.R., Essock, S.M., Becker, D.R., Wolfe, R., & Swain, K. (2004). The Hartford study of supported employment for persons with severe mental illness. *Journal of Consulting and Clinical Psychology*, *72*, 479–490.

Mueser, K.T., Salyers, M.P., & Mueser, P.R. (2001a). A prospective analysis of work in schizophrenia. *Schizophrenia Bulletin*, *27*, 281–296.

Murphy, M. (1998). Rejection, stigma, and hope. *Psychiatric Rehabilitation Journal*, *22*, 185–188.

Provencher, H., Gregg, R., Mead, S., & Mueser, K. (2002). The role of work in the recovery of persons with psychiatric disabilities. *Psychiatric Rehabilitation Journal*, *26*, 132–144.

Resnick, S., Rosenheck, R., & Lehman, A. (2004). An exploratory analysis of correlates of recovery. *Psychiatric Services*, *55*, 540–547.

Rickwood, D. (2004). *Pathways of Recovery: Preventing Relapse*. Canberra, Australia: Department of Health and Ageing.

Rogers, E.S., Anthony, W.A., Cohen, M., & Davies, R.R. (1997). Prediction of vocational outcome based on clinical and demographic predictors among vocationally ready clients. *Community Mental Health Journal*, *33*, 99–112.

Rowland, L.A., & Perkins, R.E. (1988). You can't eat, drink or make love eight hours a day: the value of work in psychiatry – a personal view. *Health Trends*, *20*, 75–79.

Rutman, I.D. (1994). How psychiatric disability expresses itself as a barrier to employment. *Psychosocial Rehabilitation Journal*, *17*, 15–35.

Spillane, R. (1999). Australian managers' attitudes to mental illness. *Journal of Occupational Health and Safety*, *15*, 359–364.

Strong, S. (1998). Meaningful work in supportive environments: experiences with the recovery process. *American Journal of Occupational Therapy*, *52*, 31–38.

Tsang, H., Lam, P., Ng, B., & Leung, O. (2000). Predictors of employment outcome for people with psychiatric disabilities: a review of the literature since the mid-80s. *Journal of Rehabilitation*, *66*, 19–31.

Van Dongen, C.J. (1996). Quality of life and self-esteem in working and non-working persons with mental illness. *Community Mental Health Journal*, *32*, 535–548.

Waghorn, G, & Chant, D. (2005) Employment restrictions among persons with ICD-10 anxiety disorders: characteristics from a population survey. *Journal of Anxiety Disorders*, *19*, 642–657.

Waghorn, G., Chant, D., & King, R. (2005a). Work-related self-efficacy among community residents with psychiatric disabilities. *Psychiatric Rehabilitation Journal*, *29*, 105–113.

Waghorn, G., Chant, D., White, P., & Whiteford, H. (2004a). Delineating disability, labour force participation and employment restrictions among persons with psychosis. *Acta Psychiatrica Scandinavica*, *109*, 279–288.

Waghorn, G, Chant, D., White, P., & Whiteford, H. (2005b). Disability, employment and work performance among persons with ICD-10 anxiety disorders. *Australian and New Zealand Journal of Psychiatry*, *39*, 55–66.

Waghorn, G., Chant, D., & Whiteford, H. (2002). Clinical and non-clinical predictors of vocational recovery for Australians with psychotic disorders. *The Journal of Rehabilitation*, *68*, 40–51.

Waghorn, G. & King, R. (1999). Australian trends in vocational rehabilitation for psychiatric disability. *Journal of Vocational Rehabilitation*, *13*, 153–163.

Waghorn, G., & Lewis, S. (2002). Disclosure of psychiatric disabilities in vocational rehabilitation. *Australian Journal of Rehabilitation Counselling*, *8*, 67–80.

Waghorn, G., Still, M., Chant, D., & Whiteford, H. (2004b). Specialised supported education for Australians with psychotic disorders. *Australian Journal of Social Issues*, *39*, 443–458.

Whooley, M.A., Kiefe, C.I., Chesney, M.A., Markovitz, J.H., Matthews K., & Hulley, S.B. (2002). Depressive symptoms, unemployment and loss of income. *Archives of Internal Medicine*, *162*, 2614–2620.

World Health Organization. (2001). *The World Health Report 2001. Mental Health: New Understanding, New Hope*. Geneva: World Health Organization.

Xie, H., Dain, B.J., Becker, D.R., & Drake, R.E. (1997). Job tenure among people with severe mental illness. *Rehabilitation Counseling Bulletin*, *40*, 230–239.

Chapter 2
EVIDENCE-BASED SUPPORTED EMPLOYMENT

Chris Lloyd

Chapter overview

Evidence suggests that most people with mental illness who receive supported employment services, such as individual placement and support, can work in a competitive employment. This chapter discusses the benefits of work, employability, barriers faced by people returning to work, different vocational approaches and evidence-based approaches. It then goes on to discuss some of the interventions that could be used to improve the outcomes attained by supported employment.

Introduction

The last two decades have seen a shift in how vocational rehabilitation is provided. Traditional vocational rehabilitation was a stepwise process that took place over time. The prevailing thought was that it was necessary to train people prior to placing them in a work situation. Typically, clients participated in group programmes, followed by long periods of assessment prior to them receiving more customised employment assistance. The evidence now supports the opposite approach (place then train) (Bond et al., 2008). The Individual Placement and Support model of supported employment is the most extensively researched model of supported employment for people with a severe mental illness. The core principles of this model are a focus on competitive employment, eligibility based on consumer choice, rapid job search, integration of mental health and employment services, attention to consumer preferences, individualised job supports and personalised benefits counselling (Bond, 2004). The purpose of this chapter is to provide a summary of competitive employment outcomes that evaluate evidence-based supported employment.

Benefits of work

Work is a basic right we all take for granted. Yet, for many people with mental illness they are excluded from this basic right. Work has many advantages for people as it provides such benefits as providing a source of social identity and status and social contacts and support; a means of structuring and occupying time, activity and involvement, and a sense of personal achievement; and importantly providing an income (Rinaldi & Perkins, 2004). People with a mental illness are sensitive to the negative effects of unemployment, for example demoralisation, loss of hope, inactivity, loss of purpose, structure, roles and status and a sense of identity (Waghorn & Lloyd, 2005). Work is very important in maintaining mental health and in promoting recovery as it enables social inclusion and meaningful participation in the wider community. Many people with mental illness identify employment as crucial to their recovery process (Provencher et al., 2002). Prolonged unemployment is linked to worsening mental health, whereas having a job can lead to reduction in symptoms, fewer hospital admissions and reduced service use (Drake et al., 1999). In addition, unemployment for people with a mental illness may lead to a range of social problems such as debt and social isolation (Social Exclusion Unit, 2004).

Employability

Individuals with psychiatric disability have the lowest rates of employment amongst all groups of people with disability (Loveland et al., 2007). It would seem from the research that individual characteristics have little impact on vocational outcomes. For example, it has been shown that there is little relationship between employment outcomes and diagnosis, severity of impairment and social skills. Nordt et al. (2007) found that higher education was connected with higher vocational status. Participants hospitalised for the first time had a higher vocational status as did previous work experience. The relative stability of vocational status and the association with years of past work experience confirmed the findings of previous research that prior employment status and work history are strong and consistent predictors of current employment status (e.g. Tsang et al., 2000).

Barriers faced by people returning to work

People with mental illness are less likely to be employed than any other group of disabled people. Workforce participation rate for people with a mental illness has been found to be 29% compared to people with physical disability (49%) and the general community (74%) (Mental Health Council of Australia, 2007). This situation is worse for people with a psychotic disorder with only 2 in 10 being in some form of employment (Mental Health Council of Australia, 2007).

Demands of the labour market, complications associated with disability benefits and limited availability of vocational rehabilitation programmes are the contributing factors (Loveland et al., 2007). It has been found that people with mental illness living in areas with high unemployment rates are less likely to be working (Becker et al., 2006). Many consumers of mental health services view the potential loss of their disability income as the primary barrier to returning to work (Loveland et al., 2007). McQuilken et al. (2003) found that most consumers in their study were working or wanted to work. However, well over half of the people agreed they could not risk losing their benefits by getting a job. This implies that many consumers who say that they are not interested in work or who are not looking for work would be interested in looking for work if they were better educated about the ways to work and make extra income, without losing all of their benefits.

Severe mental illnesses, particularly schizophrenia, are characterised by impairments in cognitive functioning and the presence of positive and negative symptoms. Cognitive deficits may include impairments in attention, working memory or problem-solving skills, and negative symptoms (e.g. apathy, social withdrawal and low energy) can undermine an individual's ability to benefit from rehabilitation services (Harvey et al., 2004; MacDonald et al., 2003). Functional limitations included social (e.g. interacting with others), emotional (e.g. managing symptoms), cognitive (e.g. assessing one's own work performance) and physical (e.g. maintaining work stamina) (MacDonald et al., 2003). Johannesen et al. (2007) found that the results of their study confirmed that having a mental illness is a critical concern for those people with severe mental illness seeking employment.

Social competence is an essential component of vocational functioning among people with severe mental illness to seeking and keeping a job (Tsang & Pearson, 1996, 2000). It has been found to be one of the most significant predictors of employment outcome (Tsang et al., 2000). Nevertheless, interpersonal difficulty was reported to be the most frequently reported job problem (58%) that led to job terminations among people with severe mental illness (Becker et al., 1998). It is mainly because they do not possess social skills necessary in the workplace (Bell & Lysaker, 1995; Lysaker et al., 1995), which in turn becomes an obstacle to their job acquisition and retention. It has been found that the more barriers to employment, the lower the likelihood of attaining employment (Johannesen et al., 2007).

Different vocational approaches

Over the years there have been a number of differing forms of vocational rehabilitation available. These are briefly described below.

Clubhouse

The clubhouse model grew from Fountain House, established in 1948, and there are now approximately 300 clubhouses in various countries around the world, which are recognised by the International Center for Clubhouse Development. Clubhouses are communities where members can achieve confidence and support to lead vocationally productive and satisfying lives. The clubhouse is organised around the work-ordered day which provides opportunities for members to contribute within a rehabilitative environment. Clubhouses assist with career development, job search and job choice (McKay et al., 2005).

Transitional employment

Transitional employment (TE) is a defining feature of clubhouse programmes and is designed to give members who lack work experience, confidence or work skills, and the opportunity to work in real jobs for real pay. The staff member provides full on-the-job training and assists the member with any issues that may arise. The main features of TE programmes are as follows: positions involve 6–9 months of temporary work, members are paid award wages, members complete the work at the employer's place of business, all work is entry level and does not require qualifications, an absence of work history and/or hospitalisation will not affect a member's chance to obtain a position, no resume or interview is required as the selection process is done by the clubhouse staff and members (Mental Health Council of Australia, 2007).

Social firms

Social firms originated in Italy in the 1960s and since then they have been found throughout Europe and the UK. They are not-for-profit businesses that provide accessible employment for people with disability. Social firms usually have the following features: dedicated between 20 and 50% of positions to employees with disability; pay all workers the award rate or productivity-based rates; provide all employees with the same employment opportunities, rights and obligations; generate the majority of their income through the commercial activity of the business (Mental Health Council of Australia, 2007).

Non-integrated pre-vocational services

Non-integrated pre-vocational services use a stepwise 'train and place' approach to vocational rehabilitation. These types of services provide vocational training covering such areas as generic work skills and personal development training in such areas as confidence building, assertiveness and stress management (Rinaldi & Perkins, 2007). In these types of programmes, participants must learn pre-vocational and work readiness skills before they are placed in work settings, which are often sheltered in that they are owned by the hospital or rehabilitation agency (Corrigan et al., 2007).

Sheltered work

Sheltered workshops were conceived for people with severe mental illness who presented a low level of functioning and who were not ready to participate in the workplace. Clients are paid according to the piece rate or achievement but the pay is usually low. Sheltered workshops create a certain type of environment where everyone has a mental illness, the work is repetitive and monotonous, and they are time-unlimited. In the past, sheltered workshops usually did factory contracts and operated in a protected and segregated environment such as a psychiatric institution (Corbiere & Lecomte, 2007).

Evidence-based approaches

Supported employment is an evidence-based psychosocial intervention for people with mental illness. Bond et al. (2001a) found the following to be the components that are predictive of better employment outcomes: the agency providing supported employment services is committed to competitive employment as an attainable goal for its clients with severe mental illness; supported employment programmes use a rapid job search approach to help clients obtain jobs directly; staff and clients find individual job placements according to client preferences, strengths and work experiences; follow-up supports are maintained indefinitely; and the supported employment programme is closely integrated with the mental health treatment programme. Together these principles serve as a foundation for evidence-based guidelines for providing effective supported employment services.

Research has shown that programmes that adhere closely to the six principles of supported employment achieve better employment outcomes (Becker et al., 2006). Specifically, mental health agencies with a higher percentage of supported employment staff per number of adults served in the community support programme provided greater access to supported employment services. It was found that agencies that fully implemented the critical components of supported employment had better outcomes (Becker et al., 2006; McGrew & Griss, 2005).

Individual Placement and Support

In particular, the Individual Placement and Support (IPS) model of supported employment has demonstrated superiority to alternative means of vocational rehabilitation for people with mental illness. Drake et al. (1996) compared supported employment services in two contrasting programmes. These included a professional rehabilitation agency outside of the mental health centre that provided pre-employment skills training and support in obtaining and maintaining jobs and an IPS model which integrated clinical and vocational services within the mental health centre. The results showed that clients in the IPS programme were more likely to be competitively employed throughout most of the 18-month follow-up. They were also more likely to work more total hours and earn more total wages. A later study by Drake et al. (1999) evaluated the effectiveness of two approaches to vocational services. Individual placement and support in which employment specialists within the mental health centre help clients to obtain competitive jobs and provide ongoing support was compared to enhanced vocational rehabilitation in which stepwise vocational services are delivered by rehabilitation agencies. During the 18-month study, it was found that participants in the IPS programme were more likely to become competitively employed (60.8% vs 9.2%) and to work at least 20 hours per week in a competitive job (45.9% vs 5.3%). The researchers concluded that the IPS model of supported employment is more effective than standard, stepwise-enhanced vocational rehabilitation approaches for achieving competitive employment, even for inner-city clients with poor work histories and multiple problems.

Lehman et al. (2002) assessed the effectiveness of the IPS model of supportive employment relative to usual psychosocial rehabilitation services for improving employment among inner-city clients with severe mental illness. Individuals in the IPS programme were more likely than the comparison group to work (42% vs 11%) and to be employed competitively (27% vs 7%). They also worked more hours and earned more. It was concluded that the IPS programme was more effective than the psychosocial rehabilitation in helping clients achieve employment goals. The researchers noted that achieving job retention remains a challenge with both interventions. Mueser et al. (2004) compared three approaches to vocational rehabilitation for severe mental illness: the IPS model of supported employment, a psychosocial rehabilitation programme and standard services. Clients in IPS had significantly better employment outcomes than clients receiving psychosocial rehabilitation and standard services, including more competitive work (73.9% vs 18.2% vs 27.5%, respectively) and any paid work (73.9% vs 34.8% vs 53.6%, respectively). The findings suggested that IPS is superior to psychosocial rehabilitation using TE as well as to brokered vocational services, including services brokered to an off-site supported employment programme.

Gold et al. (2006) designed and implemented a programme blending Assertive Community Treatment with an IPS model. In a randomised controlled trial, they compared this programme to a traditional programme providing parallel vocational and mental heath services on competitive work outcomes for adults with severe mental illness. More participants in the IPS programme held competitive jobs (64% vs 26%) and earned more income than comparison participants. It was concluded that the competitive work outcomes of this rural IPS programme closely resemble those of urban supported employment programmes. They suggested that achieving economic self-sufficiency and developing careers probably require increasing access to higher education and jobs imparting marketable technical skills. Latimer et al. (2006) aimed to determine the effectiveness of the IPS model in a Canadian setting. Participants were randomly assigned to receive either supported employment or traditional vocational services. Over the 12 months of follow-up, 47% of clients in the supported employment group obtained at least some competitive employment vs 18% of the control group. They averaged 126 hours of competitive work vs 72 in the control group. They suggested that supported employment proved more effective than traditional vocational services in a setting significantly different from settings in the USA, and may therefore be generalised to settings in other countries.

Burns et al. (2007) conducted a randomised controlled trial in six European centres to assess the effectiveness of the IPS programme. They were able to show the effectiveness of IPS in a widely differing labour market and welfare context. Burns et al. (2007) suggested that this service was an effective approach for vocational rehabilitation in mental health. Bond et al. (2007) conducted a randomised controlled trial which compared two vocational models (IPS and diversified placement approach). They found that IPS was superior to the diversified placement approach in achieving vocational outcomes. They concluded that IPS is more effective for helping people with mental illness achieve competitive employment outcomes than a psychiatric rehabilitation approach. Bond et al. (2001b) found that clients who worked in competitive employment for an extended period of time showed a greater rate of improvement in several non-vocational outcomes, for example a reduction in psychiatric symptoms, satisfaction with vocational services, leisure and finances and in self-esteem.

In a study conducted by Wong et al. (2008), they examined the effectiveness and applicability of a supported employment programme based on the individual placement and support model in a Hong Kong setting. Over the 18-month study period, as compared with participants in the conventional vocational rehabilitation programme, those in the supported employment were more likely to work competitively (70% vs 29%), held a greater number of competitive jobs, earned more income, worked more days and sustained longer job tenures. They found that consistent with previous research findings in the USA, the supported employment programme was more effective than the conventional vocational rehabilitation programme in helping individuals with long-term mental illness find and sustain competitive employment in a Hong Kong setting. Killickey et al. (2008) examined whether IPS was a useful intervention for those with first-episode psychosis. It was found that the IPS group had significantly better outcomes on level of employment, hours worked per week, jobs acquired and longevity of employment. The IPS group also significantly reduced their reliance on welfare benefits. It was concluded that IPS had a good potential to address the problem of vocational outcome in people with first-episode psychosis. It was suggested that a co-located, early intervention approach to vocational rehabilitation might be a more useful approach than brokered employment services.

Twamley et al. (2008) examined employment outcomes among middle-aged and older participants with schizophrenia or schizoaffective disorder in a 12-month randomised controlled trial comparing two work rehabilitation programmes: IPS and conventional vocational rehabilitation. Compared with conventional vocational rehabilitation, IPS resulted in statistically better work outcomes, including attainment of competitive employment, number of weeks worked and wages earned. Participants who obtained competitive employment reported improved quality of life over time compared with those who did not. Age was not significantly associated with attainment of competitive work. They suggested that more knowledge is needed regarding how to best help clients overcome barriers to employment, for example fear of losing benefits, lack of confidence and lack of transportation.

Interventions to improve supported employment

A variety of interventions that directly improve employment outcomes could be used to augment supported employment. These are discussed below firstly at a service level and then as individual interventions.

Implement and disseminate supported employment programmes

Vocational rehabilitation programmes significantly improve the employment rates of individuals with mental illness. Supported employment has been found to be more effective than other vocational rehabilitation programmes at helping people with a mental illness overcome barriers to employment. In establishing IPS services it may well help to impart to the care team a practical understanding of the evidence base, in particular the evidence on client characteristics, the likely predictors of relapse and the need to encourage all clients to participate, regardless of their job readiness or individual problems (Rinaldi et al., 2008).

Integration of supported employment

Research has demonstrated that closer coordination between clinical and vo-cational services leads to better employment outcomes for people with severe mental illness (Bond et al., 2001b). It has been found that clients who re-ceived integrated services attained higher rates of employment, more hours of employment and higher wages from competitive employment than clients who received non-integrated services. Drake et al. (2003) found that systems that integrate mental health and vocational services through multidisciplinary teams appear to have several advantages including a greater capacity to engage and retain individuals in services, better communication between disciplines, changing the philosophy of the mental health system about the importance of work in the recovery of people with mental illness and developing more effective vocational service plans that take clinical considerations into account. Cook et al. (2005) found that when clinical and vocational staff worked together in multidisciplinary teams at the same location using a unified case record and meeting together regularly, participants were more likely to work competitively and work 40 hours or more per month. The results of this study confirm the importance of provider communication and the coordination of psychiatric and rehabilitation services in working towards vocational goals.

Improving the fidelity of supported employment

Bond et al. (2002) suggest that the use of fidelity scales is an essential component of evidence-based practice. Fidelity scales measure the degree of implementation of a practice, that is, the degree of attainment of practice standards. The Supported Employment Fidelity Scale (SE Fidelity Scale) is a 15-item telephone-administered instrument measuring fidelity of supported employment for people with mental illness. Each item is rated on a five-point behaviourally anchored scale, with a score of 5 indicating full implementation, 4 indicating moderate implementation and the remaining scale points indicating increasingly larger departures from the standards of supported employment. The items assess structural elements of programme implementation in the domains of staffing, organisation and services (Bond et al., 2008). The 15 items are summed to give a total score ranging from 15 to 75. A score greater than 65 is regarded as high fidelity, while a score of 65 or lower is considered as low fidelity. Any score below 56 is an absence of fidelity, that is, very low fidelity. In a study examining supported fidelity ratings at baseline and every 6 months thereafter, it was found that all sited achieved fidelity within 1 year, and most of the improvements in fidelity were achieved during this initial period (Bond et al., 2008).

Augmenting supported employment with supported education

Supported education is a promising intervention which can help individuals meet the demands of the labour force. There are a variety of models of supported education, including skills training, classrooms on campus, group support on campus and community-based models. Results have been encouraging in that most studies have found improvements in self-confidence, cognitive functioning and completion of college courses for people receiving supported education (Collins et al., 1998). Given that many people with a psychotic disorder may well have developed the illness at a critical time of maturation, this has the potential to disrupt education and career planning. It is important to pay attention to the educational needs of people with a mental illness who are wishing to work. Killickey et al. (2008) found that the courses undertaken by individuals with first-episode psychosis were in keeping with vocational objectives, for example a licence or certificate for employment required in the participant's desired area of work. (See Chapter 12 for more information on supported education.)

Increase access to benefits counselling

People with a mental illness fear losing benefits. Increasing access to benefits counselling is another intervention that has been shown to improve income levels for individuals with mental illness (Tremblay et al., 2004). Ongoing planning and guidance to help clients make well-informed decisions regarding social security, health insurance and other government entitlements is important (Bond, 2004). Benefits counselling assists the participant to develop and plan to manage his or her benefits through the transition to employment. Tremblay et al. (2004) suggest firstly to undertake benefits screening in order to verify the participant's current benefits status and determining what benefits issues might impact the participant's employment goals. The next step is explaining to the participant how employment would impact the benefits he or she receives and assisting the participant to make informed choices based on this information. This also includes helping the participant to take advantage of the various work incentives that are available. The final step is benefits management, which is the process of assisting the participant to develop and implement a plan to manage his or her benefits through the transition to employment.

Skills training

To improve vocational outcomes from IPS, various enhanced versions have been developed by augmenting IPS with additional psychosocial interventions. Skills training techniques include a variety of delivered strategies that individuals can use to help manage and cope with the symptoms of their psychiatric condition, reduce their susceptibility to relapse and improve their adaptive functioning in life. Skills training strategies usually consist of highly structured, manualised interventions that may include psychoeducation, behavioural interventions, cognitive techniques or a combination of interventions (Loveland et al., 2007). Tsang (2001), in a pilot study, showed that the social skills training module together with appropriate professional support afterwards is effective in enhancing the social competence and vocational outcomes for people with a mental illness. Participants first received training on verbal and non-verbal communication, accurate social perception, assertiveness, grooming and personal appearance, greetings and other basic conversation skills. Afterwards, they proceeded to the core work-related skills including those required for job searches, phone and face-to-face interviews, social skills in specific situations in the workplace such as handling conflicts and requesting sick leave and also problem-solving skills. The module was translated into different languages and was found to be effective in other countries such as Germany (Roder et al., 2006). An Integrated Supported Employment programme (ISE; Tsang, 2003) was developed, which combines IPS with work-related social skills training. A randomized controlled trial has shown that more ISE participants became competitively employed and worked longer than IPS (Tsang et al., 2009).

Conclusions

People with mental illness would like to work. Vocational rehabilitation aims to assist clients with this goal. Over the years there have been a number of different model proposed. The model of supported employment, in particular the IPS, has demonstrated superiority in vocational outcomes for people with a mental illness. This chapter has reviewed the outcomes of applying this model and has found that there have been very good results with people on the whole earning more income, working more days and sustaining longer job tenures. However, there is still the problem with people maintaining their employment over time. There are a number of interventions that could be used to augment supported employment. These have been addressed firstly as a service wide approach, which is then followed by some more individually tailored interventions.

References

Becker, D.R., Drake, R.E., Bond, G.R., Xie, H., Dain, B.J., & Harrison, K. (1998). Job termination among persons with severe mental illness participating in supported employment. *Community Mental Health Journal, 34,* 71–82.

Becker, D.R., Xie, H., McHugo, G.J., Halliday, J., & Martinez, R.A. (2006). What predicts supported employment program outcomes? *Community Mental Health Journal, 42,* 303–313.

Bell, M.D., & Lysaker, P.H. (1995). Psychiatric symptoms and work performance among people with severe mental illness. *Psychiatric Services, 46,* 508–510.

Bond, G.R. (2004). Supported employment: evidence for an evidence-based practice. *Psychiatric Rehabilitation Journal, 27,* 345–359.

Bond, G.R., Becker, D.R., Drake, R.E., Rapp, C.A., Meisler, N., Lehman, A.F., Bell, M.D. & Blyler, C.R. (2001a). Implementing supported employment as an evidence-based practice. *Psychiatric Services, 52,* 313–322.

Bond, G.R., Campbell, K., Evans, L.J., Gervey, R., Pascaris, A., Tice, S., Del Bene, D., & Revell, G. (2002). A scale to measure quality of supported employment for persons with severe mental illness. *Journal of Vocational Rehabilitation, 17*, 239–250.

Bond, G.R., McHugo, G.J., Becker, D.R., Rapp, C.A., & Whitley, R. (2008). Fidelity of supported employment: lessons learned from the national evidence-based practice project. *Psychiatric Rehabilitation Journal, 31*, 300–305.

Bond, G.R., Resnick, S.G., Drake, R.E., Xie, H., McHugo, G.J., & Bebout, R. B. (2001b). Does competitive employment improve nonvocational outcomes for people with severe mental illness? *Journal of Counseling and Clinical Psychology, 69*, 489–501.

Bond, G.R., Salyers, M.P., Dincin, J., Drake, R.E., Becker, D.R., Fraser, V.N., & Haines, M. (2007). A randomized controlled trial comparing two vocational models for persons with severe mental illness. *Journal of Consulting and Clinical Psychology, 75*, 968–982f.

Burns, T., Catty, J., Becker, T., Drake, R.E., Fioretti, A., Knapp, M., Lauber, C., Rossler, R., Tomov, T., van Busshbach, J., White, S., & Wiersma, D. (2007). The effectiveness of supported employment for people with severe mental illness: a randomized controlled trial. *Lancet, 370*, 1146–1152.

Collins, M.E., Bybee, D., & Mowbray, C.T. (1998). Effectiveness of supported education for individuals with psychiatric disabilities: results from an experimental study. *Community Mental Health Journal, 34*, 595–613.

Cook, J.A., Lehman, A.F., Drake, R., McFarlane, W.R., Gold, P.B., Leff, H.S., Blyler, C., Toprac, M.G., Razzano, L.A., Burke-Miller, J.K., Blankertz, L., Shafer, M., Pickett-Schenk, S.A., & Grey, D.D. (2005). Integration of psychiatric and vocational services: a multisite randomized, controlled trial of supported employment. *American Journal of Psychiatry, 162*, 1948–1956.

Corbiere, M., & Lecomte, T. (2007). Vocational services offered to people with severe mental illness. *Journal of Mental Health, 16*, 11–13.

Corrigan, P.W., Larson, J.E., & Kawabara, S.A. (2007). Mental illness stigma and the fundamental components of supported employment. *Rehabilitation Psychology, 52*, 451–457.

Drake, R.E., Becker, D.R., Bond, G.R., & Mueser, K.T. (2003). A process analysis of integrated and non-integrated approaches to supported employment. *Journal of Vocational Rehabilitation, 18*, 51–58.

Drake, R.E., McHugo, G.J., Anthony, W.A., & Clark, R.E. (1996). The New Hampshire study of supported employment for people with severe mental illness. *Journal of Consulting and Clinical Psychology, 64*, 391–399.

Drake, R.E., McHugo, G.J., Bebout, R.R., Becker, D.R., Harris, M., Bond, G.R., & Quimby, E. (1999). A randomised clinical trial of supported employment for inner-city patients with severe mental disorders. *Archives of General Psychiatry, 56*, 627–633.

Gold, P.B., Meisler, N., Santos, A.B., Carnemolla, M.A., Williams, O.H., & Keleher, J. (2006). Randomized trial of supported employment integrated with assertive community treatment for rural adults with severe mental illness. *Schizophrenia Bulletin, 32*, 378–395.

Harvey, P.D., Green, M.F., Keefe, R.S.E., & Velligen, D.I. (2004). Cognitive functioning in schizophrenia: a consensus statement on its role in the definition and evaluation of effective treatments for the illness. *Journal of Clinical Psychiatry, 65*, 361–372.

Johannesen, J.K., McGrew, J.H., Griss, M.E., & Born, D. (2007). Perceptions of illness as a barrier to work in consumers of supported employment services. *Journal of Vocational Rehabilitation, 27*, 39–47.

Killickey, E., Jackson, H.J., & McGorry, P.D. (2008). Vocational intervention in first-episode psychosis: individual placement and support v. treatment as usual. *British Journal of Psychiatry, 193*, 114–120.

Latimer, E.A., Lecomte, T., Becker, D.R., Drake, R.E., Duclos, I., Piat, M., Lahaie, N., St-Pierre, M.S., Therrien, C., & Xie, H. (2006). Generalisability of the Individual Placement and Support model of supported employment: results of a Canadian randomised controlled trial. *British Journal of Psychiatry*, *189*, 65–73.

Lehman, A.F., Goldberg, R., Dixon, L.B., McNary, S., Postrado, L., Hackman, A., & McDonnell, K. (2002). Improving employment outcomes for persons with severe mental illnesses. *Archives of General Psychiatry*, *59*, 165–172.

Loveland, D., Driscoll, H., & Boyle, M. (2007). Enhancing supported employment services for individuals with a serious mental illness: a review of the literature. *Journal of Vocational Rehabilitation*, *27*, 177–189.

Lysaker, P., Bell, M., Sito, W.S., & Bioty, S.M. (1995). Social skills at work: deficits and predictors of improvement in schizophrenia. *Journal of Nervous and Mental Disease*, *183*, 688–692.

MacDonald, K.L., Rogers, E.S., & Massaro, J. (2003). Identifying relationships between functional limitations, job accommodations, and demographic characteristics of persons with psychiatric disabilities. *Journal of Vocational Rehabilitation*, *18*, 15–24.

McGrew, J.H., & Griss, M.E. (2005). Concurrent and predictive validity of two scales to assess the fidelity of implementation of supported employment. *Psychiatric Rehabilitation Journal*, *29*, 41–47.

McKay, C., Johnsen, M., & Stein, R. (2005). Employment outcomes in Massachusetts clubhouses. *Psychiatric Rehabilitation Journal*, *29*, 25–33.

McQuilken, M., Zahniser, J.H., Novak, J., Starks, R.D., Olmos, A., & Bond, G.R. (2003). The work project survey: consumer perspectives on work. *Journal of Vocational Rehabilitation*, *18*, 59–68.

Mental Health Council of Australia (2007). *Let's Get to Work. A National Mental Health Employment Strategy for Australia*. Melbourne: Mental Health Council of Australia.

Mueser, K.T., Clark, R.E., Haines, M., Drake, R.E., McHugo, G.J., Bond, G.R., Essock, S.M., Becker, D.R., Wolfe, R., & Swain, K. (2004). The Hartford study of supported employment for persons with severe mental illness. *Journal of Consulting and Clinical Psychology*, *72*, 479–490.

Nordt, C., Muller, B., Rossler, W., & Lauber, C. (2007). Predictors and course of vocational status, income, and quality of life in people with severe mental illness: a naturalistic study. *Social Science and Medicine*, *65*, 1420–1429.

Provencher, H.L., Gregg, R., Mead, S., & Mueser, K. T. (2002). The role of work in the recovery of persons with psychiatric disability. *Psychiatric Rehabilitation Journal*, *26*, 132–144.

Rinaldi, M., & Perkins, R. (2004). Vocational rehabilitation. *Psychiatry*, *3*, 54–56.

Rinaldi, M., & Perkins, R. (2007). Comparing employment outcomes for two vocational services: Individual Placement and Support and non-integrated pre-vocational services in the UK. *Journal of Vocational Rehabilitation*, *27*, 21–27.

Rinaldi, M., Perkins, R., Glynn, E., Montibeller, T., Clenaghan, M., & Rutherfrod, J. (2008). Individual Placement and Support: from research to practice. *Advances in Psychiatric Treatment*, *13*, 50–60.

Roder, V., Muller, DR., & Zorn, P. (2006). Social skills training in vocational rehabilitation of schizophrenia patients: advantages of work-related social skills training in comparison to unspecific social skills training. *Zeitschrift für Klinische Psychologie und Psychotherapie*, *35*, 256–266.

Social Exclusion Unit. (2004). *Mental Health and Social Exclusion*. Wetherby, UK: ODPM Publications.

Tsang, H., Lam, P., Ng, B., & Leung, O. (2000). Predictors of employment outcome for people with psychiatric disabilities: a review of the literature since the mid '80s. *Journal of Rehabilitation, 66,* 19–31.

Tsang, H.W.H. (2001). Applying social skills training in the context of vocational rehabilitation for people with schizophrenia. *Journal of Nervous and Mental Disease, 189,* 90–98.

Tsang, H.W.H. (2003). Augmenting vocational outcomes of supported employment by social skills training. *Journal of Rehabilitation, 69*(3), 25–30.

Tsang, H.W.H., Chan, A., Wong, A., & Liberman, R.P. (2009). Vocational outcomes of an integrated supported employment program for individuals with persistent and severe mental illness. *Journal of Behavior Therapy and Experimental Psychiatry, 40,* 292–305.

Tsang, H.W.H., & Pearson, V. (1996). A conceptual framework for work-related social skills in psychiatric rehabilitation. *Journal of Rehabilitation,* July/August/September, 61–66.

Tsang, H.W.H., & Pearson, V. (2000). Reliability and validity of a simple measure for assessing the social skills of people with schizophrenia necessary for seeking and securing a job. *Canadian Journal of Occupational Therapy, 67,* 250–259.

Tremblay, T., Xie, H., Smith, J., & Drake, R. (2004). The impact of specialized benefits counseling services on social security administration disability beneficiaries in Vermont. *Journal of Rehabilitation, 70,* 5–11.

Twamley, E.W., Narvaez, J.M., Becker, D. R., Bartels, S.J., & Jeste, D.V. (2008). Supported employment for middle-aged and older people with schizophrenia. *American Journal of Psychiatric Rehabilitation, 11,* 76–89.

Waghorn, G., & Lloyd, C. (2005). The employment of people with mental illness. *Australian e-journal for the Advancement of Mental Health, 4*(2,Suppl.)

Wong, K.K., Chiu, R., Tang, B., Mak, D., Liu, J., & Chiu, S.N. (2008). A randomised controlled trial of a supported employment program for persons with long-term mental illness in Hong Kong. *Psychiatric Services, 59,* 84–90.

Chapter 3

THE SUCCESSES AND CHALLENGES OF INTEGRATING MENTAL HEALTH AND EMPLOYMENT SERVICES

Samson Tse and Nikki Porteous

Chapter overview

The most effective form of client-centred employment services for people with the experience of serious mental illness is the Individual Placement and Support (IPS) approach (Bond, 1998). In New Zealand this evidence-based supported employment model has been implemented successfully. In this chapter we reflect on the barriers of accessing supported employment services for clients of mental health services. These include the institutional, individual and other barriers. The delivery of vocational services in New Zealand adopts three basic formats: parallel mode, attachment mode of supported employment service and fully integrated mode of IPS approach of supported employment service. Our IPS case study is 'WorkFirst', which has been implemented in Wellington, New Zealand. The context-specific benefits, what it looks like in practice, formative evaluation, fidelity scale, learning and reflections are discussed.

Introduction

Earlier approaches to vocational rehabilitation assumed that people with mental illness would never be ready to work or if they would, they need a prolonged period of time for assessment, training and preparation before being placed in a real job for real pay. Nevertheless, research shows that in most settings about 75% of persons with mental illness want to work (Corrigan et al., 2008). There is a genuine desire among people with personal experience of mental illness to re-enter the labour market for financial reason, for self-fulfillment or for facilitating a more active social life. 'First and foremost I'd like to be stabilized . . . with this and then I would like to go to college or something . . . you know I'd like to get back to work eventually (Anita). I hope to work, you know, get a job and work. 'Cos I mean there's no life without a job, which is true (Jai)' (users' narratives, cited in Cohen, 2008, p. 162).

Over the past 15 years, an integrated approach to supported employment has demonstrated strong evidence of success in supporting individuals who are impaired by a mental illness to secure paid employment (for comprehensive reviews on supported employment, see Corrigan et al., 2008, and Rosen & Barfoot, 2001). The remaining challenge is to provide evidence-based employment services by fully integrating employment and mental health services.

Consistent with numerous independent studies on the effectiveness of the IPS model of supported employment, Catty et al. (2008) reported that the IPS service was more effective than usual vocational rehabilitation services based on the 'train and place' model for every vocational outcome (e.g. number of working days, duration of the longest held position), in a multi-site randomised controlled trial located in six European centres: London, Ulm–Günzburg, Rimini, Zurich, Groningen and Sofia. On the basis of the sample of 312 participants in the study, they also found that previous work history was the only client characteristic predictive of all employment outcomes and unmet social needs were associated with higher probability of working in competitive employment. Remission in the first 6 months of the study period was related to obtaining paid positions but was not predictive of getting a job subsequently. Furthermore, there were two intriguing findings concerning the relationships between the clients and professionals or between vocational workers and characteristics of the employment services which were not assessed in previous clinical trials. Firstly, the client–vocational worker relationship (such as understanding of the clients' needs, commitment to helping the clients) was found to be predictive of securing competitive employment regardless of the services that the research participants were randomly allocated to. Secondly, if the service models were removed from the analysis, it was found that the shorter time gap to enter the vocational service was associated with working for more hours in open employment. 'This was because time to service entry was confounded by service type, with IPS services being more likely to take patients on more swiftly: in fact, all but two IPS patients were taken into the services by T_1 (*first 6 monthsof the study period*)…' (Catty et al., 2008, p. 229, italics added).

Providing individuals with the experience of mental illnesses with quick and immediate access to vocational services – be it IPS or usual vocational service available in local mental health services – is not a new challenge. Twenty years ago, McCrory wrote in one of the classic texts on vocational rehabilitation: 'Vocational rehabilitation services *have usually been considered late*, if at all, in the treatment process. By then, the client has accepted the "chronic patient" role, and he and his family have adapted their expectations to his impaired state' (McCrory, 1988, p. 209, italics added).

This chapter sets out to explore to what extents the vocational rehabilitation services are integrated with mental health services to ensure that clients have swift access to specialised vocational support services. The chapter concludes by examining an example of integrating mental health and employment services in Wellington, New Zealand.

Table 3.1 Barriers faced by service users in accessing supported employment services.

Institutional barriers	Individual barriers	Other barriers
• Stigma and discrimination associated with mental illness • Lack of confidence in clients' ability to work in competitive employment • Lack of services options • Lack of flexibility	• Lack of awareness of the availability of supported employment services • Lack of self-esteem/self-confidence • Lack of hope • Confusion about benefit or income support	• Lack of positive role model • Lack of transport

Barriers in accessing evidence-based supported employment service

Regardless of the fact that an evidence-based IPS model of practice is emerging and is increasingly available in most developing countries, users of mental health services are still facing a variety of barriers in accessing a much-needed vocational rehabilitation service (Table 3.1).

Barriers can be classified into three major levels: institutional, individual and other barriers. With regards to institutional barriers, Peterson et al. (2004) found 34% of participants in the New Zealand national survey reported being discriminated against by mental health services, which was higher than general health services (23%). Stigma is the status loss and discrimination is unfair treatment triggered by negative stereotypes about individuals labelled as mentally ill. 'People with a mental illness are among the most socially and economically marginalised members of the community' (Waghorn & Lloyd, 2005, p. 1).

Closely related to stigma and discrimination evident in some mental health services is the lack of belief at an institutional level in users' potential to return to the labour market. Some mental health services offer limited options of supported employment services. Sadly, service users have to adjust their expectations and fit themselves to existing services and not vice versa. Another illustration of institutional barrier is about how the services are being delivered, for example having rigid hours of services, insistence on disclosure of mental health history and limited provision of follow-up services. With regards to individual level of barriers, it might be that service users have limited knowledge and information about types of supported employment services available in the local area. A sense of confidence and positive self-esteem is critical to enable individuals affected by mental illness not only to articulate their vocational aspirations and access employment services, but also to navigate through often a very complex health care system.

Hope is very critical to recovery; it is a multidimensional concept which reflects an interaction of a person's thoughts, feelings, actions and relationships (Anthony, 1993; Deegan, 1988; Russinova, 1999). Without a sense of hope about what one can accomplish vocationally, it is unlikely that a service user will access supported employment services. It is well documented that welfare money or income support may become a disincentive for individuals to work or contemplate pursuing any vocational goals. With regards to other barriers, the lack of positive role models or inspiration from service users 'who have been there and done that' may diminish an individual's interest in accessing supported employment. Finally, in practical terms, without transport assistance some clients may have little motivation to seek support from employment services.

Service delivery context

The present authors argue that, provided that an IPS model of supported employment is delivered in an appropriate context, most of these barriers in accessing employment services could be removed. Corrigan et al. (2008) outlined seven principles of evidence-based supported employment. They include:

(1) Clients, not the professionals, should make decisions about their readiness to participate in supported employment services
(2) Provision of counselling on benefit or income support so that clients can make good decisions about vocational goals and aspirations
(3) Clients' preferences regarding vocational goals, type of work, working setting, hours, supports and timing, and disclosure of mental illness should be acknowledged and taken into consideration when planning employment service
(4) Assessment and training is minimised, instead the client should be supported to rapidly pursue a job of the client's choice
(5) Follow-along support service is available for as long as the client requires them
(6) Supported employment service is most effective and efficient when it is supported by a multidisciplinary team
(7) Integration of employment and mental health services at all levels is paramount so that clients can gain the maximum benefit from mental health care service. 'At the local level, vocational rehabilitation counselors join mental health teams to ensure that services are individually tailored and take advantage of the expertise and resources of both agencies' (Corrigan et al., 2008, p. 198).

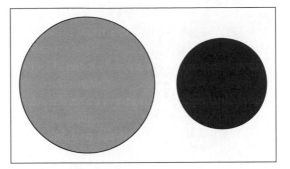

Figure 3.1 Parallel mode of delivery. Grey circle denotes mental health service and dark circle denotes supported employment service.

Broadly speaking, there are three forms of integration between employment and mental health services, namely parallel, attachment and integration mode of delivery.

Parallel mode of delivery

The clinical team and supported employment service are based at different geographical locations or different parts of the mental health and social service (Figure 3.1). Supported employment workers do not attend clinical meetings; their involvement is merely on the 'as-required' basis. Referrals are initiated to the supported employment service after members of the clinical team have performed screening on the clients and have determined who may benefit from the supported employment service or may receive direct referrals from clients themselves. In some cases, they may receive funding from different sources (e.g. Ministry of Social Development vs Ministry of Health) and are accountable for different sets of organisational values and goals as well.

Attachment mode of delivery

Supported employment workers are invited or expected to attend clinical meetings on a regular basis (Figure 3.2). Supported employment workers and the clinical team discuss and decide which clients will benefit from supported employment services. Although the attachment mode of delivery is likely the most common form of collaboration between employment and mental health services in outpatient or community teams, it remains unclear if this form of service system is the most productive platform to facilitate the IPS integrated mode of supported employment. There are three major limitations of the attachment mode of delivery:

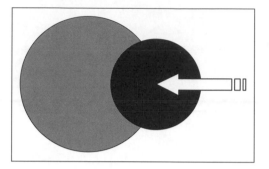

Figure 3.2 Attachment mode of delivery. Grey circle denotes mental health service and dark circle denotes supported employment service.

(1) Vocational workers tend to restrict their involvement to the time when they are attending multidisciplinary team meetings, whereas a lot of clinical discussions often take place outside formal meetings.

(2) Given the vocational workers are brought into the clinical team from outside, vocational rehabilitation may be seen as 'tag on' or even luxury service.

(3) Vocational workers may not see themselves as part of the team and do not necessarily give full attention to the clients under their care, especially when they are carrying a heavy caseload from other services.

Integrated mode of delivery

Ideally the IPS workers are co-located together with the clinical team in the same physical address to achieve maximum integration between employment and mental health service where vocational targets and aspirations become completely integrated with traditional treatment outcomes and goals (Figure 3.3). Employment becomes part of the initial assessment, the treatment plan,

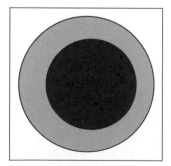

Figure 3.3 Integrated mode of delivery. Grey circle denotes mental health service and dark dotted circle denotes Individual Placement and Support approach of supported employment service.

the services delivery package, and the outcomes review process for *every client who has a vocational goal*' (Corrigan et al., 2008, p. 198, italics added). As such, a client's entry to the supported employment service will virtually take no extra effort on the part of the client and multidisciplinary team. IPS workers are in very close communication with members of the multidisciplinary team to provide comprehensive rehabilitation service. A fully integrated recovery orientated mental health service is characterised by:

(1) Comprehensive service including supported employment is available for each service user who wants or needs it
(2) A standardised intervention process is guided by the user's outcomes rather than the particular professional's area of expertise
(3) Referrals between an array of services includes clear statements of user's outcomes expected of service providers
(4) Policies and systems encourage the development and implementation of integration strategies to achieve specific user's outcomes (Anthony, 2006; for discussion on client-centred, recovery-oriented service, see Anthony, 2006, pp. 340–357 and Adams & Grieder, 2005). Dr Norman Sartorius, who is the Director of the Division of Mental Health at the World Health Organization added, 'Goals of rehabilitation of people who have had a mental illness are changing and so are the principles that govern them ... It is likely that, in the future, rehabilitation will no longer be the task of health and social services: it has to become a *joint enterprise of these services* and people who have mental impairments and their families' (Sartorius, 2002, p. 219, italics added).

Case study

Context

In 2000–2001, a pilot IPS service was developed at Capital & Coast District Health Board's (C&CDHB) Early Intervention Service (EIS). This is a specialist community mental health team assessing and treating 13–25-year-olds for their first episode of a psychotic illness. For marketing purposes, the service was branded 'WorkFirst' and the occupational therapist's role changed from generic care management and specific key work to that of employment consultancy.

In 2002, WorkFirst became one of four providers nationally with the Ministry of Social Development's (MSD's) demonstration project, named 'employable'. This 2-year contract enabled WorkFirst to recruit a second employment consultant in a consumer role. The results were not published but vocational outcomes and feedback from clients and clinicians resulted in a second 2-year contract with the MSD between 2004 and 2006. A larger, third, 2-year contract followed, and currently WorkFirst's revenue comes from the partner-ship between C&CDHB and MSD.

At the time of writing, WorkFirst has six employment consultants integrated with five of C&CDHB's community mental health teams. Three of the staff members are occupational therapists including the coordinator and three are non-clinicians with bachelor degrees or equivalent, plus the relevant experience in the delivery of mental health or disability sector services. Consumers or people with personal experience of mental illness are encouraged to apply for these positions.

Specific benefits

WorkFirst was developed in response to the unmet vocational needs of the clients receiving treatment from the EIS. Transition from school to study is a developmental step for this age group and a mental illness often disrupts this (Cattermole, 1995; Dougherty et al., 1996). As an occupational therapist in a primarily generic role with a care management caseload, N.P. (the second chap-ter author) did not have enough time to provide the intensive level of support re-quired to assist clients into work and study. Employment services are often inad-equate to meet the special needs of this client group. It fitted with the 'one-stop-shop' approach of the service, providing more assertive and intensive psychoso-cial rehabilitation to prevent clients from developing chronic mental illness.

The health benefits of being meaningfully occupied in paid employment or enrolled in study have been well documented. In the EQOLISE trial of IPS in Europe, Burns et al. (2007) found that those working were significantly less likely to be rehospitalised and that IPS doubles the access to work of people with psychotic illnesses without evidence of increased relapse. The cost benefits to health are therefore also evident.

A person moving off social welfare benefits and into employment plus paying taxes has cost benefits for MSD and the government. With unemployment low and labour shortages high, the MSD were able to shift their focus from unemployed beneficiaries to those dealing with sickness and invalids benefits.

What does the integrated approach look like in practice?

Adhering to the principles of IPS or evidence-based supported employment, WorkFirst is fully integrated with the clinical community mental health teams (see Figure 3.3). The employment consultants are members of the multidis-ciplinary teams and peers of their clinical colleagues. They are employees of C&CDHB. They sit at desks in the same office and attend the multidisciplinary team meetings. They hold no clinical responsibilities such as care management or duty, but practise full-time in their employment consultancy roles and are well supported by their clinical colleagues to do so.

Each employment consultant has a caseload of up to 25 clients or jobseekers. Referrals are mostly from their clinical colleagues, with the only criteria being an expressed desire to work or study by the client. They can choose from the following interventions offered:

- Career planning and development
- CV writing
- Job-seeking skills
- Preparation for job interview
- Course information
- Disclosure counselling
- Sources of funding
- Marketing to employers
- Ongoing support

To assist with marketing to employers, WorkFirst has branded itself with business cards and flyers which do not identify the employment consultants as working from a mental health service. Unmarked cars are used to prevent the IPS workers from being identified as employees of C&CDHB. Training in marketing and selling is provided to every employee who wears the appropriate dress code for the role. WorkFirst offers free assistance to employers by:

- Providing employees ready for work
- Job matching
- Job retention
- Return to work after a period of illness
- Ongoing support
- Access to wage subsidies or other funding

Employment consultants find that most jobseekers prefer not to disclose they have a mental illness to employers due to fear of discrimination. This limits the consultant's ability to become familiar with their employment situation, meet their employer and support them in work. Employment consultants also experience employer's discrimination when attempting to market to employers and disclosing that the jobseeker has a history of mental illness. Therefore, WorkFirst is inclined to market more discretely.

Disclosure also occurs on occasions when a client who is working becomes unwell and the employer has to give them leave from work. Employment law protects the job, as it is illegal to dismiss an employee on the grounds of ill-health. This then becomes an opportunity for the employment consultant to liaise with the employer, assist with job retention and a return to work. Respect for the client's confidentiality is adhered to by consulting with the client as to what information they feel comfortable in sharing with the employer.

As the WorkFirst team is located in different community mental health teams on separate locations in the Wellington C&CDHB region, it is important that the employment consultants can communicate with each other on a regular basis. They meet weekly for business, group supervision, service development and journal club where staff members share learning, resources and expertise. Each staff member receives individual supervision fortnightly. As an organizational member of the Association Supported Employment New Zealand, each employment consultant can access opportunities for training with them and attend their annual conference.

Listen and learn: What do service users, practitioners and employers say?

The following examples of quotes from clients reflect their views of WorkFirst:

- 'Your one is way better (than the vocational service as usual). It's easier and way quicker'.
- 'You helped but *I did it on my own*' (italics added).
- 'If it wasn't for the flat and the job I would probably have self harmed more and who knows what could have happened. I haven't done anything stupid now for like five weeks or so. I have lost count'.

Clinicians say:

- 'You offer something quite different that talking clinicians don't always offer. *Hope*' (italics added).
- 'You are easily accessible. I like the immediacy of dialogue and you are there'.
- 'This sort of work is essential in any effective contemporary community mental health service. Without employment or vocational study, many people loose a sense of meaning and role, which in turn impacts adversely on mental health, and may even be a prime determinant of wellbeing.'.

An employer:

- 'There are definite advantages in having a consultant to support employees who need it. They were very focused in finding the "right" placement, and were positive'.

A disability coordinator and tutor on campus:

- 'I couldn't fault this service. Highly skilled, highly experienced, good facilitators, absolutely top of the line. It's not a job for anyone with little experience'.

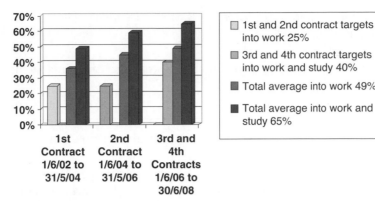

Figure 3.4 Results of evaluation to date.

• 'WorkFirst communicated well with the student, provider and other agencies, were committed and reliable, available with a team approach, which are important factors for a service like this'.

Formative evaluation

WorkFirst receives some funding from MSD. A contract obligation is to provide bimonthly reports that give an account of participant numbers and outcomes to MSD. The service has consistently exceeded contract targets (Figure 3.4). In the first 4 years of funding, the contract target was 25% into work. Initially, WorkFirst achieved over 30%, and then over 40% by the fourth year. In the next two years of funding, the contract target was 40% into work and study. WorkFirst exceeded this target again. After 6 years of service delivery the overall outcomes have averaged 49% into work and 65% into work and study.

Systematic study is required to examine the application of IPS in New Zealand context and further development for this type of service delivery in New Zealand and internationally.

Fidelity scale

WorkFirst has used the Supported Employment Fidelity Scale – Implementation Questions (Becker et al., 2001) to assess the quality of evidence-based employment service implementation and the extent of fidelity to the IPS approach. Scores between 66 and the maximum 75 on this scale indicate good fidelity of implementation of the IPS approach. In December 2007, each employment consultant in each of the four teams scored it independently, and then the scores were collated and independently overseen by a researcher. Overall, WorkFirst was scored 69/75, reflecting good fidelity implementation.

High implementation was scored on 8 of the 15 items. These included the following eight items:

(1) *Caseload size*: Employment specialists manage caseloads of up to 25 clients.
(2) *Exclusively vocational*: Employment specialists provide only vocational services.
(3) *Generalist model*: Each employment specialist carries out all phases of vocational services.
(4) *Contact with mental health team*: Employment specialists are part of Mental Health Treatment Teams; they routinely share decision-making with this team.
(7) *Continuous assessment:* Vocational assessment is ongoing and based on work experiences in competitive jobs.
(9) *Client choice:* Client preferences and needs determine employer contracts, not the job market.
(10) *Diversity of jobs:* Jobs diverse in type and setting.
(12) *Multiple jobs:* Clients are assisted in finding new jobs after employment ends.

The remaining seven items helped employment consultants to identify the challenges of implementation, which resulted in some strategies to overcome these challenges:

(5) *Vocational unit:* Employment specialists work as a unit – have group supervision and shared caseloads.
   Strategy: As work consultants work from different bases in different parts of the geographical region, the consultants are now meeting weekly rather than fortnightly in order to work more closely together. As a consequence, caseloads are now shared more with group supervision, and on occasions the consultants cover clients from their caseloads when on leave from work.
(6) *Zero exclusion:* No eligibility requirements (such as job readiness) for programme.
   Strategy: Zero exclusion as resulted in referrals for clients who are pre-ferring not to seek for paid employment or study immediately, but just want something to do. An introduction to WorkFirst is very helpful to introduce them to the idea that paid employment or study is an option and when they are ready they can access us for this type of support.
(8) *Rapid search:* Job search occurs rapidly after programme entry.
   Strategy: One of the staff was finding it a challenge to implement rapid search. A need for more targeted supervision and training was identified.
(11) *Permanent jobs:* Jobs are competitive and permanent.

Strategy: As not all jobs attained are permanent, this scored us down on the scale but the consultants felt that the item did not reflect the labour market or the terms of the MSD contract, whereby 'continuous' jobs where a person remains off the benefit is counted as sustainable.

(13) *Follow along:* Individualised, time-unlimited support provided to employers and clients.

Strategy: This item is not always easy to achieve when the client is discharged from the clinical team in which the employment consultant works. If ongoing support is required, the consultants facilitate referrals to non-government organisation providers of supported employment.

(14) *Community based:* Vocational services are provided in the community.

Strategy: Proportionally less of the consultants' time is spent in the community than what is recommended on the scale. The consultants feel it is because a large number of clients do not want to disclose to employers that they experience mental illness, which means that the consultants' support is more in the background than at the work place. As the consultants work individually with clients in a large urban region, and due to the limitations imposed by not disclosing, the consultants do not market the service widely to employers in the region. However, it has made the IPS workers reflect on the issue of disclosure and possibly more towards the 'managing personal information' approach, that is to normalise the sharing of any visible signs of functional impairment (e.g. working at a slower pace, difficulty in concentration) in everyday language that may require workplace accommodations.

(15) *Assertive outreach:* Assertive outreach when needed.

Strategy: The staff members based in the adult community mental health teams use this approach less than those working from the early intervention psychosis and youth specialty teams. Once again the need to address this in supervision and with in-service training was identified.

When implementing this scale the employment consultants could see the advantage of developing our own New Zealand scale, which would better reflect the unique New Zealand culture, the New Zealand labour market, consumer participation in service delivery, the different employment and educational needs of adolescents, and the increased use of information technologies.

Learning and reflections

Initially, establishing this IPS in a First Episode Psychosis specialist community mental health team has been one reason for its success. The principles of IPS fit very well with the principles of First Episode Psychosis, as they both provide early, intensive, assertive and client-centred practices. The other C&CDHB

mental health services have been able to observe this and then enthusiastically incorporate IPS into their teams when the opportunity arose.

Practicing as employment consultants, their roles are *solely vocational with no clinical role or tasks*. This has largely been well supported by clinical team leaders and colleagues who value the employment consultants' roles and experience first-hand the beneficial effects that WorkFirst has on clients' recovery.

The presence of employment consultants in the teams has resulted in '*enhanced care management*'. In consultation with the employment consultants and having access to the appropriate resources, the clinicians are more mindful of the employment status of their clients and will perform some employment-related tasks. These may include assistance with CVs, job search and monitoring the clients' performance in work or study.

WorkFirst initially created a 'consumer employment consultant' role to be explicit in its intent to recruit and promote *consumer participation and service delivery*. WorkFirst has learned to recruit people with the necessary qualifications, skills and experience to meet the requirements of the job being consistent with the other staff, rather than just because they are consumers. WorkFirst now feels that having 'consumer' in the title may detract some potential applicants as it plays too large an emphasis on the consumer part of the role. When recruiting for any position, WorkFirst is now encouraging all potential applicants with the experience of mental illness to apply. Practising as an employment consultant integrated with the clinical team is an opportunity for more service users to be service providers, provides positive role models for clients and assists with the engagement of clients with services.

Occupational therapists have a key role in the development, delivery, promotion and coordination of evidence-based supported employment (Porteous & Waghorn 2007; Porteous & Waghorn, 2009). Occupational therapists understand the value that life roles and meaningful occupations have on a person's well-being and recovery from mental illness. Other mental health professions with an enthusiasm for this type of service delivery are just as able to fulfill this role as well.

WorkFirst also practices *supported education*. Working with youth, the employment consultants recognise that transition from school to tertiary study is often interrupted by their mental illness. WorkFirst also acknowledges that higher qualifications lead to more satisfying careers and better pay in the long run. The MSD is prepared to recognise this, enabling us to work equably with clients regardless of whether they want work or study or both.

The non-clinical staff members have short-term contracts, as their positions are reliant on the receipt of continued funding from MSD. As a result they have no *career pathway* and do not receive pay parity with their clinical colleagues. As this challenges their loyalty to the service, it also impacts on staff retention. As a result, WorkFirst is attempting to align employment consultants on the same collective employment agreement and salary bands as their clinical peers.

Having a supported employment service integrated with the clinical mental health services assists with the *engagement of clients* with these services. A client may not be identifying a need for medical treatment but may want a job. This one-stop-shop approach demonstrates to clients that the mental health service is able to assist them in a multitude of ways depending upon what the clients want.

Increasingly, the employment consultants have found a need for *return to work and job retention* services within the teams. One of the employment consultants is spending half-a-day per week on the adult acute psychiatric in-patient ward to provide an early intervention approach to job retention and return to work for those admitted acutely that they want to keep their jobs.

C&CDHB's regional *forensic service* has recognised a need for employment consultancy to meet the unmet employment needs of clients referred from forensic psychiatric service. As a result, a WorkFirst position has been created there, integrated with the forensic community mental health team. This will provide new challenges by working with some high profile forensic clients and managing the added stigma of a mental illness plus a criminal history.

Conclusions

In the past few years, it has been encouraging to see the development of IPS services internationally and particularly in New Zealand and Australia. There is no right or wrong way to establish IPS services, just the right service delivery principles to adhere to and the services are adequately funded. Consistently, in surveys clients say that what they want is work. The results of a recent survey titled as the 'Knowing the People Planning' (King & Welsh, 2006) identified that occupation is the greatest unmet need among people with enduring mental illness in New Zealand. In that survey, both clients and clinicians indicated that the best indicator of recovery is for a person to be in regular paid employment where possible.

Future studies are needed to examine the context in which integration is most needed, and specific intervention strategies that are most effective. Inclusion of fidelity test is another priority research area to ensure that the IPS model of supported employment delivered in different contexts (e.g. adolescent mental health versus forensic mental health services) is providing services in a manner consistent with their articulated theory. Lastly, more studies are required to promote the generalisability of the evidence internationally, given all of the studies on delivery of the IPS model of supported employment services were conducted in English-speaking and European countries, coupled with variation in the nature of the health service system.

References

Adams, N., & Grieder, D.M. (2005). *Treatment Planning for Person-Centered Care: The Road to Mental Health and Addiction Recovery.* Burlington, MA: Elsevier Academic Press.

Anthony, W.A. (1993). Recovery from mental illness: the guiding vision of the mental health services system in the 1990s. *Psychosocial Rehabilitation Journal, 16,* 11–23.

Anthony, W.A. (2006). A recovery-oriented service system: setting some system-level standards. In: Davidson, L., Harding, C., & L. Spaniol, L. (eds) *Recovery from Severe Mental Illnesses: Research Evidence and Implications for Practice,* Vol. 2. Boston: Boston University, Center for Psychiatric Rehabilitation, pp. 340–357.

Becker, D.R., Smith, J., Tanzman, B., Drake, R.E., & Tremblay, T. (2001). Fidelity of supported employment programs and employment outcomes. *Psychiatric Services, 52,* 834–836.

Bond, G. (1998). Principles of the Individual Placement and Support model: empirical support. *Psychiatric Rehabilitation Journal, 22,* 11–23.

Burns, T., Catty, J., Becker, T., Drake, R.E., Fioretti, A., Knapp, M., Lauber, C., Rossler, R., Tomov, T., van Busshbach, J., White, S., & Wiersma, D. (2007). The effectiveness of supported employment for people with severe mental illness: a randomized controlled trial. *Lancet, 370*(9593), 1146–1152.

Cattermole, T. (1995). Transitional homes programme: supported education and employment programme. *Community Mental Health in New Zealand, 9,* 31–34.

Catty, J., Lissouba, P., White, S., Becker, T., Drake, R.E., Fioritti, A., Knapp, M., Lauber, C., Rossler, W., Tomov, T., van Busschbach, J., Wiersma, D., & Burns, T. (2008). Predictors of employment for people with severe mental illness: results of an international six-centre randomised controlled trial. *British Journal of Psychiatry, 192,* 224–231.

Cohen, B. MZ (2008). *Mental Health User Narratives: New Perspectives on Illness and Recovery.* New York: Palgrave MacMillan.

Corrigan, P.W., Mueser, K.T., Bond, G.R., Drake, R.E., & Solomon, P. (2008). *Principles and Practice of Psychiatric Rehabilitation: An Empirical Approach.* New York: The Guilford Press.

Deegan, P. (1988). Recovery: the lived experience of rehabilitation. *Psychosocial Rehabilitation Journal, 11,* 11–19.

Dougherty, S.J., Campana, K.A., Kontos, R.A., Flores, M.K.D., Lockhart, R.S., & Shaw, D.D. (1996). Supported education: a qualitative study of the student experience. *Psychiatric Rehabilitation Journal, 19,* 59–70.

King, D., & Welsh, B. (2006). *Knowing the People Planning (KPP): A New, Practical Method to Assess the Needs of People with Enduring Mental Illness and Measure the Results.* London: The Nuffield Trust. Available at: www.kpp.org.nz (accessed 5 November 2008).

McCrory, D.J. (1988). The human dimension of the vocational rehabilitation process. In: Ciardiello, J.A., & Bell, M.D. (eds) *Vocational Rehabilitation of Persons with Prolonged Psychiatric Disorders.* Baltimore, MD: The Johns Hopkins University Press, pp. 208–218.

Peterson, D., Pere, L., Sheehan, N., & Surgenor, G. (2004). *Respect Costs Nothing: A Survey of Discrimination Faced by People with Experience of Mental Illness in Aotearoa New Zealand.* Auckland: Mental Health Foundation.

Porteous, N., & Waghorn, G. (2007). Implementing evidence-based employment services in New Zealand for young adults with psychosis: progress during the first five years. *British Journal of Occupational Therapy, 70,* 521–526.

Porteous, N., & Waghorn, G. (2009). Developing evidence-based supported employment services for young adults receiving public mental health services. *New Zealand Journal of Occupational Therapy*, 56, 34–39.

Rosen, A., & Barfoot, K. (2001). Do day care and occupation: structured rehabilitation and recovery programmes and work. In: Thornicroft, G., & Szmukler, G. (eds) *Textbook of Community Psychiatry*. New York: Oxford University Press, pp. 295–308.

Russinova, Z. (1999). Providers' hope-inspiring competence as factor optimizing psychiatric rehabilitation outcomes. *Journal of Rehabilitation*, 65, 50–57.

Sartorius, N. (2002). *Fighting for Mental Health: A Personal View*. Cambridge, UK: Cambridge University Press.

Waghorn, G., & Lloyd, C. (2005). The employment of people with mental illness. *Australian e-Journal for the Advancement of Mental Health* 4(2), 1–43.

Chapter 4

REDUCING EMPLOYERS' STIGMA BY SUPPORTED EMPLOYMENT

Hector W.H. Tsang, Mandy W.M. Fong, Kelvin M.T. Fung and Patrick W. Corrigan

Chapter overview

Work is a significant factor of mental health and contributes remarkably to the rehabilitation and recovery of people with mental illness. Unemployment has been extensively documented as detrimental to mental health (Catalano et al., 2000; Fryer, 1997; Hammarstroem & Janlert, 1997; Schaufeli, 1997; Warr et al., 1988). Work not only improves financial situation, but also provides daily structure and routine and meaningful goals. Individuals with employment possess a sense of personal well-being, self-efficacy and social identity (Siu et al., in press). It improves self-esteem and self-image, reduces symptom levels, promotes social contacts as well as facilitates quality of life of those individuals (Ackerman & McReynolds, 2005; Becker et al., 2005; Bond et al., 2001; Morgan, 2005).

Barriers to employment

Although work is demonstrated to be of great significance to mental health, the employment rate among people with mental illness is unacceptably low (Anthony et al. 2002; Equal Opportunities Commission, 1997; Rosenheck et al., 2006). Research has revealed that most individuals with mental illness have the desire to work (Bates, 1996; Hatfield et al., 1992; Rinaldi & Hill, 2000; Sainfort et al., 1996; Secker et al., 2001; South Essex Service User Research Group, Secker, & Gelling, 2006). The discrepancy between the above is due to the presence of individual and environmental barriers that block individuals' return to competitive employment. Individuals with mental illness encounter various personal and environmental challenges. At the personal level, many of them have low educational attainment, low productivity, poor work history, poor social and work-related skills, negative and cognitive symptoms, medication side effects and lack of work experience (Anthony & Jansen, 1984; Cook, 2006; Fabian, 1992; Ferdinandi et al., 1998). In addition, barriers to getting employment at the environmental level include unfavourable labour market dynamics, lack of appropriate vocational and clinical services, ineffective work incentive programmes, work disincentives, labour force discrimination and public stigma (Cook, 2006; Henry & Lucca, 2004; Marwaha & Johnson, 2004; Tsang et al., 2003). Environmental barriers not only constituted a hurdle for individuals with mental illness to gainful employment; it also exerted a negative impact on the individuals' beliefs and thus self-efficacy. In response to public stigma, individuals with mental illness might internalise the negative stereotypes from the public, which resulted in demoralised personal qualities and impeded self-esteem (Fung et al., 2007). This self-stigma is believed to further affect individuals' recovery and employment (Corrigan et al., 2006; Fung et al., 2007; Ritsher & Phelan, 2004; Vauth et al., 2007) as they might act against themselves (Corrigan & Watson, 2002). They may eventually adopt withdrawal and avoidant coping behaviours (Bandura, 1986; Fung et al., 2007; Vauth et al., 2007).

Since stigma in fact is one of the most important barriers to gainful employment among individuals with mental illness (Schulze & Angermeyer, 2003; Surgeon General, 2000), the stigmatising attitudes of employers and co-workers towards them are particularly important (Link, 1987; Stuart, 2006; Tsang et al., 2007). Studies showed that individuals with mental illness who have already obtained competitive employment may quit their work as a result of the workplace stigma and interpersonal difficulties (Mak et al., 2006; Stuart, 2006). Individuals may experience discrimination at the workplace when their mental illness is revealed (Stuart, 2006). The co-workers would demonstrate their reluctance to associate with them and become judgemental (Peterson et al., 2006). In this chapter, we first discuss the stigma employers hold towards individuals with mental illness and then the types of steps we can take to diminish this so as to facilitate their employment.

Employer stigma

Goffman (1963) defined stigma as the mark that distinguishes someone as discredited. People marked by skin colour (ethnicity), physiology (gender), body size (obesity) and clothes (poverty) are stigmatised by the general public. There is ample evidence showing the presence of labour force discrimination (Bordieri & Drehmer, 1986; Diksa & Rogers, 1996; Farina & Felner, 1973; Link, 1982, 1987; Olshanksy et al., 1960; Wahl, 1999; Webber & Orcutt, 1984). Some studies suggested that discrimination of employment resulted from employers' negative attitudes towards mental illness (Feldman, 1988; Manning & White, 1995; Rochlin, 1987; Thomas et al., 1993; Wilgosh & Skaret, 1987), which in turn reflected broader societal views that people with mental illness are incompetent and dangerous (Pescosolido et al., 1999). To use Jorm's terminology, these stigmatising attitudes may be conceptualised as a problem of limited mental health literacy or an inability to appropriately recognise mental disorders as treatable illnesses (Jorm, 2000; Jorm et al., 1997). In the hiring context, this mental health illiteracy prompts the employer to inaccurately judge the abilities and employability of employees with psychotic disorders. Although applying stereotypes about mental illness to all people with mental illness is problematic, some research suggests that stereotypes may possess a 'kernel of truth'. Employers who encounter an applicant with mental illness may accurately judge that these individuals may, for example, have excessive absenteeism or cognitive disturbances that impede work performance. On the other hand, the unilateral application of this reasoning (an increased likelihood of problematic performance) to every case represents the crux of discrimination and may have harmful consequences for the applicant (Tsang et al., 2007).

Discrimination from employers towards mental illness is the most commonly cited barrier to gaining employment (Rinaldi & Hill, 2000). A questionnaire surveyed a sample of 200 personnel directors of public companies and found that half of the respondents never or only occasionally hired someone who was currently mentally ill (Manning & White, 1995). Their response fell to 28% when they were asked about hiring people who were previously ill. People with schizophrenia were more likely to be dismissed if they became ill while in their position when compared to those with other types of mental illness. More than 80% of employers believed individuals being sick for a physical illness. However, the figure was only 63% as to mental illness. Interestingly, larger companies were found to be significantly more likely to hire people with mental illness. It is suggested that larger companies may have more resources that could be able to accommodate employees with mental illness (Marwaha & Johnson, 2004).

In order to provide various kinds of assistance to employers for reducing their stigmatising attitudes towards people with mental illness, we need to have a better understanding of their specific concerns about hiring these individuals. There is emerging evidence that employers had many negative beliefs relating to hiring individuals with mental illness. Some studies showed that employers had worries about their work performance, work personality and symptoms (Diksa & Rogers, 1996; Johnson et al., 1988). Employers expressed concerns on their poor quantity and quality of work, brief tenure, absenteeism and low flexibility. Previous studies also showed that the concerns included the need for additional supervision, taking little pride in work, low acceptance of work role, difficulty following instructions, poor ability to socialise and low work persistence. Other studies showed that employers also carried negative beliefs about people with mental illness to the personal level (Cook et al., 1994; Hand & Tryssenaar, 2006) that included low motivation to work, low work quantity, likelihood of injury, problem in following directions, being unable to make friends and poor anger management. On the other hand, employers expressed that providing accommodation for employees with mental illness would create difficulty from much to extreme (Combs & Omvig, 1986).

A significant body of evidence showed that employers showed less willingness to hire individuals with mental illness due to their dangerousness, reduced productivity and the presence of strange behaviours (Feldman, 1988; Rochlin, 1987; Thomas et al., 1993; Tsang et al., 2007; Wilgosh & Skaret, 1987). A study by Tsang et al. (2007) interviewed 100 employers from six industries that included manufacturing, education, health services, high and low technology businesses across three cities – Chicago, Beijing and Hong Kong – and found that employers were concerned about the safety threat posed to the co-workers and customers, productivity and job performance, strange and unpredictable behaviours, and the potential for relapse. Perception of safety threat to the public constitutes the main reason for stigmatising behaviours. Literature reveals that psychotic disorders were historically segregated from society because they were considered dangerous (Brockington et al., 1993; Cohen & Struening, 1962; Link et al., 1999; Taylor & Dear, 1981). As stated by Johnson-Dalzine et al. (1996), perceptions of dangerousness may directly lead to fear. Given these concerns, employers are likely to reject an applicant with an acknowledged psychotic disorder. Since the study was conducted in different cities of different cultures, it also examined the cultural difference in employers' concerns about hiring people with mental illness. Among the four expressed concerns, employers across the three cities expressed most consistently that they were concerned about the compromised job performance and productivity. Although the perception of dangerousness is found to be one of the most common stereotypes relating to mental illness (Pescosolido et al., 1999), the study found that employers in Hong Kong were more concerned about it than those in Beijing and Chicago, which may be accounted for by the tendency of the media and press in Hong Kong to exaggerate the crime and violent behaviours committed by people with psychotic disorders (Tsang et al., 2007). Moreover, employers in Hong Kong and Beijing, though to a lesser extent, were more likely to indicate their concerns about the strange and erratic behaviours of employees with mental illness. The study further compared Chinese and American employers and found that Chinese employers were more likely to view employees with mental illness so as to demonstrate a weaker work ethic and less loyalty to their companies. Another interesting finding is that employers in Hong Kong and Beijing tended to rank such 'soft skills' as trustworthiness, work motivation and ability to relate to others more importantly than did Chicago employers. Similarly, many of the Chinese employers' concerns about hiring people with psychotic disorders related to issues such as interpersonal volatility and negative impact of the psychotic worker on the other employees. One interpretation of this difference is that the Chinese employers' heightened concern reflects the collectivistic and interdependent nature of the Chinese culture due to the practice of Confucian values (King & Bond, 1985; Pearson, 1995). Confucianism originated from China, which can be viewed as a social ethic, a political ideology and a scholarly tradition (Tu, 1998). The Confucian believes that harmony is an essential element for the peaceful life of people, family and states (Yao, 2000). Individuals are expected to shape their life to realise harmony (Yao, 2000). The deviant behaviour of mental illness is regarded as the absence of moral standard, and it would violate the harmonious social relationship expected by Confucianism (Tsang et al., 2007). In addition, people with severe mental illness create enormous shame to the family, which affect the reputation of the family (Tsang et al., 2007). In Western societies, employers in this study were less likely to express concerns about whether employees get along with others compared to their concerns that employees possess the requisite skills to accomplish the job. In Chinese communities, collectivistic values are manifested in employers' concerns about their relationships with the supervisor, co-workers and customers. An illustration of this cross-cultural difference is concerns about health and smoking. Employers in Chicago were not concerned whether the employee is healthy or whether he or she smokes. However, employers in Hong Kong and Beijing were more concerned about health issues in the workplace and their effects on other people and the image of the company. On the other hand, employers in Chicago were more concerned about disorganised thoughts that might interfere with their ability to follow instructions and get things done (Scheid, 2005). Thus, this is suggested that the concerns of employers in China tended to be more people-oriented, while the expressed concerns of employers in the USA were more task-oriented.

Steps to overcome employers' stigma

Given the recent recognition of employment barriers experienced by people with mental illness and the need for providing of evidence-based practices to overcome these barriers, studies on the development of vocational rehabilitation services to assist people with mental illness in becoming successfully employed have been mushrooming (Ackerman & McReynolds, 2005; Tsang et al., 2009). These studies focused on minimising the impact of personal (e.g. lack of job and social skills) and/or environmental (e.g. lack of job opportunities and stigma) barriers. The rehabilitation professionals would use effective strategies and develop effective programmes to combat the workplace barriers experienced by people with mental illness. The following section therefore discusses the main types of strategies to combat stigma and the effectiveness of these strategies.

Types of anti-stigma strategies

Due to the devastating effects of stigma on gainful employment and recovery among people with mental illness, stigma reduction has recently become a major concern in psychiatric rehabilitation. It has been suggested that protest, education and contact are the three approaches to diminish the stigmatising attitudes of the public towards individuals with mental illness (Corrigan et al., 2001; Corrigan & O'Shaughnessy, 2007).

Research from social psychology has suggested that protest campaigns would possibly suppress the stigmatising attitudes and thoughts toward mental illness and behaviours that promote these attitudes. Protest is usually administered against stigmatising public beliefs, media reports and advertisements. This strategy works on conveying messages on stopping to report inaccurate representations of mental illness as well as stopping to believe negative views about mental illness. It is found to be effective in reducing negative public images of mental illness (Wahl, 1995). However, there is a potential drawback related to this strategy. A rebound effect may be observed in the stigmatising beliefs of the public (Corrigan et al., 2001; Macrae et al., 1994). Instead of diminishing stigma, people, who were ordered to suppress negative stereotypes, may after a while show more stigmatising beliefs than before (Macrae et al., 1994). Thus, although protest may be effective in reducing the stigmatisation of public images of mental illness, there is little evidence that it is effective in changing people's prejudice about mental illness. Moreover, it may also be less effective in promoting positive attitudes, as 'just say no to negative stereotypes' efforts were not demonstrated to lead people to a more enlightened thinking towards mental illness (Corrigan, 2004; Corrigan & O'Shaughnessy, 2007).

Education seeks to replace stigmatising attitudes with accurate conceptions about the illness, which is regarded as another strategy to diminish stigma of people with mental illness (Corrigan et al., 2001; Rusch et al., 2005). The change in stigma is achieved by challenging the inaccurate stereotypes and myths of mental illness (e.g. people with mental illness are not productive at work) with facts (e.g. most of them who receive vocational rehabilitation will gain a successful work outcome) (Corrigan & O'Shaughnessy, 2007). Studies have revealed that people who seem to be more knowledgeable about mental illness are less likely to endorse stigma and discrimination (Link & Cullen, 1986; Link et al., 1987; Roman & Floyd, 1981). Studies on graduate students who attended brief courses on mental illness provided evidence for the improvement in attitudes about people with mental illness (Keane, 1991; Morrison, 1980; Morrison et al., 1980; Morrison & Teta, 1980). Other various educational approaches, such as short-information sessions (Penn et al., 1994, 1999) and semester-long courses on severe mental illness (Holmes et al., 1999), have also demonstrated their effectiveness in improving attitudes of the public after their completion of the courses. However, when used alone, the effect and duration of the change in attitudes were shown to be temporary (Corrigan et al., 2001, 2002) and correlated to the pre-education programme knowledge of individuals (Holmes et al., 1999). Recent research is to combine the use of the educational approach with other strategies.

Among the three approaches for stigma reduction, contact is considered to be the most promising way in alleviating public stigma, which facilitates interaction between the public and people with mental illness (Corrigan & O' Shaughnessy, 2007). Research on racial stereotypes provided evidence that contact with people of a stigmatised group is an effective way for reducing intergroup prejudice (Desforges et al., 1991). It is reported that the general public showed significant, long-lasting improvement in their attitudes and related behavioural changes when they interact with people with mental illness (Corrigan et al., 2001, 2003). The strategy is found to be more effective when it is targeted towards a discrete power group (Fiske, 1993). In the context of reducing workplace stigma, it is suggested that contact is a good means for reducing workplace stigma (Corrigan et al., 2007).

Use of supported employment as an integrated stigma strategy

Individual Placement and Support (IPS) is an evidence-based supported employment (SE) approach for people with severe mental illness. Overseas (Bond et al., 2008) and local (Tsang et al., 2009; Wong et al., 2006) studies demonstrated its effectiveness on short-term employment. A review (Bond et al., 2008) on the randomised controlled trial of 11 high-fidelity IPS programmes suggested that employability was achieved with 61% of participants with severe mental illness, with the average job tenure for 24.2 weeks. In Hong Kong, Wong et al. (2006) revealed that 64.2% of individuals with severe mental illness obtained competitive employment after participating in the IPS programme. Their mean competitive working duration was 19.84 weeks.

Lack of social competence and social skills necessary in the workplace obstructs individuals with severe mental illness to find and keep a job (Cheung et al., 2006; Tsang, 2003; Tsang & Pearson, 2001). Thus, Tsang et al. (2009) have integrated the work-related social skills training into the IPS programme in further enhancing the employment outcomes of individuals with severe mental illness in Hong Kong. This augmented approach enabled 78.8% participants competitively employed with the job tenure lasting for 23.84 weeks. The enhancement of employment outcomes was probably due to their improved job interviewing skills and their ability to solve interpersonal difficulties in workplace (Tsang et al., 2009). The cues of mental illness among the individuals with severe mental illness may be hidden once they are able to demonstrate appropriate interpersonal skills (Schumacher et al., 2003) to reduce their likelihood to experience workplace stigma. Individuals tend to better cope with stigmatising social situations in the workplace, which then acts as a protective factor to prolong their job tenure. Besides, the employers and the co-workers may establish better attitudes towards individuals with severe mental illness through daily contacts. Positive contact experiences at the workplace may help reduce stigma and contribute to more positive attitudes towards mental illness among employers and co-workers. Moreover, SE provides meaningful work experiences, which help them increase their sense of purposefulness and

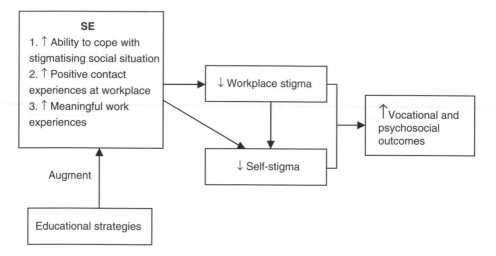

Figure 4.1 The hypothetical relationship between SE, workplace and self-stigma, and vocational and psychosocial outcomes of individuals with severe mental illness.

motivation as well as enhance their coping of mental illness stereotypes (Bryson & Bell, 1999), leading to the reduction of self-stigma (Siu et al., in press). Thus, SE programmes provide positive contact experiences between individuals with severe mental illness and employers and co-workers, which may help reduce workplace stigma.

The stigma reduction effect of SE may be amplified by educational elements provided by employment specialists. Empirical findings suggested that the public showed improved attitudes towards individuals with severe mental illness after engaging in short information sessions (Penn et al., 1994, 1999; Thornton & Wahl, 1996) or semester-long courses on psychiatric disabilities (Holmes et al., 1999). The dissemination of positive information about mental illness could be facilitated by using pamphlets, books and videos (Rusch et al., 2005; Tanaka et al., 2003). The employment specialists should incorporate these therapeutic ingredients in the SE programmes when they negotiate and discuss with the employers on the work arrangement for the clients. The relationship between SE, workplace and self-stigma, and vocational and psychosocial outcomes is illustrated in Figure 4.1.

Although individuals with severe mental illness hope to lead normal lives to enjoy meaningful works (Becker & Drake, 1994), some of them may be reluctant to pursue competitive employment due to their self-demoralisation or self-perceived incompetence (Corrigan, 2004; Fung et al., 2007; Vauth et al., 2007). This is especially common for self-stigmatised individuals to adopt withdrawal and avoidant coping behaviours (Fung et al., 2007; Vauth et al., 2007). Participating in a meaningful work experience actually help individuals with severe mental illness to increase their sense of purposefulness and motivation as well as enhance their coping of mental illness stereotypes (Bryson & Bell, 1999). Their affirmation of personal ability through work should successfully lead to an establishment of positive sense of self in combating self-stigmatisation (Siu et al., in press; Yip, 2005). Supported employment provides a context in which the clients experience success and sense of competence, which in turn will help them reduce their self-stigma and thus improve their sense of self-efficacy and personal well-being (Siu et al., in press).

Although the potential of SE as a stigma reduction tool is tremendous, it seems that there has not been any empirical attempt to evaluate its effect on reducing employers' stigma and thus exert a positive impact on their hiring practices towards people with mental illness. Researchers and clinicians should therefore target their future efforts towards better utilisation of SE as a strategy of educating employers and reducing their stigma towards people with mental illness.

References

Ackerman, G.W., & McReynolds, C.J. (2005). Strategies to promote successful employment of people with psychiatric disabilities. *Journal of Applied Rehabilitation Counseling, 36*, 35–40.

Anthony, W.A., Cohen, M., Farkas, M.D., & Gagne, C. (2002). *Psychiatric Rehabilitation*, 2nd edn. Boston: Center for Psychiatric Rehabilitation.

Anthony, W.A., & Jansen, M.A. (1984). Predicting the vocational capacity of the chronically mentally ill: research and implications. *American Psychologist, 39*, 537–544.

Bandura, A. (1986). The explanatory and predictive scope of self-efficacy theory. *Journal of Social and Clinical Psychology, 4*, 359–373.

Bates, P. (1996). Stuff as dreams are made on. *Health Service Journal, 33*, 5497.

Becker, D.R., & Drake, R.E. (1994). Individual Placement and Support: a community mental health center approach to vocational rehabilitation. *Community Mental Health Journal, 30*, 193–206.

Becker, D.R., Drake, R.E., & Naughton, W.J. (2005). Supported employment for people with co-occurring disorders. *Psychiatric Rehabilitation Journal, 28*, 332–338.

Bond, G.R., Drake, R.E., & Becker, D.R. (2008). An update on randomized controlled trials of evidence-based supported employment. *Psychiatric Rehabilitation Journal, 31*, 280–290.

Bond, G.R., Resnick, S., Drake, R.E., Xie, H., McHugo, G., & Bebout, R. (2001). Does competitive employment improve non-vocational outcomes for people with severe mental illness? *Journal of Consulting and Clinical Psychology, 69*, 489–501.

Bordieri, J.E., & Drehmer, D.E. (1986). Hiring decisions for disabled workers: looking at the cause. *Journal of Applied Social Psychology, 16*, 197–208.

Brockington, I.F., Hall, P., Levings, J., & Murphy, C. (1993). The community tolerance of the mentally ill. *British Journal of Psychiatry, 162*, 93–99.

Bryson, G.J., & Bell, M.D. (1999). Quality of life benefits if paid work activity in schizophrenia. *Schizophrenia Research, 36*, 323.

Catalano, R., Aldrete, E., Vega, W., Kolody, B., & Aguilar-Gaxiola, S. (2000). Job loss and major depression among Mexican Americans. *Social Science Quarterly*, *81*, 477–487.

Cheung, L.C.C., Tsang, H.W.H., & Tsui, C.U. (2006). A job-specific social skills training program for people with severe mental illness: a case study for those who plan to be a security guard. *Journal of Rehabilitation*, *72*, 14–23.

Cohen, J., & Struening, E.L. (1962). Opinions about mental illness in the personnel of two large hospitals. *Journal of Abnormal and Social Psychology*, *64*, 349–360.

Combs, I.H., & Omvig, C.P. (1986). Accommodation of disabled people into employment: perceptions of employers. *Journal of Rehabilitation*, *52*, 42–45.

Cook, J.A. (2006). Employment barriers for persons with psychiatric disabilities: update of a report for the president's commission. *Psychiatric Services*, *57*, 1391–1405.

Cook, J.A., Razzano, L.A., Straiton, D.M., & Ross, Y. (1994). Cultivation and maintenance of relationships with employers of people with psychiatric disabilities. *Psychosocial Rehabilitation Journal*, *17*, 103–116.

Corrigan, P.W. (2004). How stigma interferes with mental health care. *American Psychologist*, *59*, 614–625.

Corrigan, P.W., Larson, J.E., & Kuwabara, S.A. (2007). Mental illness stigma and the fundamental components of supported employment. *Rehabilitation Psychology*, *52*, 451–457.

Corrigan, P.W., Markowitz, F.E., Watson, A.C., Rowan, D., & Kubiak, M.A. (2003). An attribution model of public discrimination towards persons with mental illness. *Journal of Health and Social Behavior*, *44*, 162–179.

Corrigan, P.W., & O'Shaughnessy, J.R. (2007). Changing mental illness stigma as it exists in real world. *Australian Psychologist*, *42*, 90–97.

Corrigan, P.W., River, L., Lundin, R.K., Penn, D.L., Uphoff-Wasowski, K., Campion, J., Mathiesen, J., Gagnon, C., Bergman, M., Goldstein, H., & Kubiak, M.A. (2001). Three strategies for changing attributions about severe mental illness. *Schizophrenia Bulletin*, *27*, 187–195.

Corrigan, P.W., Rowan, D., Green, A., Lundin, R.K., River, P., Uphoff-Wasowski, K., White, K., & Kubiak, M.A. (2002). Challenging two mental illness stigmas: personal responsibility and dangerousness. *Schizophrenia Bulletin*, *28*, 293–310.

Corrigan, P.W., & Watson, A.C. (2002). The paradox of self-stigma and mental illness. *Clinical Psychology: Science and Practice*, *9*, 35–53.

Corrigan, P.W., Watson, A.C., & Barr, L. (2006). The self-stigma of mental illness: implications for self-esteem and self-efficacy. *Journal of Social and Clinical Psychology*, *25*, 875–884.

Desforges, D.M., Lord, C.G., Ramsey, S.L., Mason, J.A., Van Leeuwen, M.D., West, S.C., & Lepper, M.R. (1991). Effects of structured cooperative contact on changing negative attitudes toward stigmatized social groups. *Journal of Personality and Social Psychology*, *60*, 531–544.

Diksa, E., & Rogers, E.S. (1996). Employer concerns about hiring persons with psychiatric disability: results of the employer attitude questionnaire. *Rehabilitation Counseling Bulletin*, *40*, 31–44.

Equal Opportunities Commission. (1997). *Full Report: A Baseline Survey on Employment Situation of Persons with a Disability in Hong Kong*. Hong Kong: Equal Opportunities Commission.

Fabian, E.S. (1992). Longitudinal outcomes in supported employment: a survival analysis. *Rehabilitation Psychology*, *37*, 23–36.

Farina, A., & Felner, R.D. (1973). Employment interviewer reactions to former mental patients. *Journal of Abnormal Psychology, 82*, 268–272.

Feldman, D. (1988). Employing physically and mentally impaired employees. *Personnel, 65*, 14–15.

Ferdinandi, A., Yootanasumpun, V., Pollack, S., & Bermanzohn, P. (1998). Rehab rounds: predicting rehabilitation outcome among patients with schizophrenia. *Psychiatric Services, 49*, 907–909.

Fiske, S.T. (1993). Controlling other people: the impact of power on stereotyping. *American Psychologist, 48*, 621–628.

Fryer, D. (1997). International perspectives on youth unemployment and mental health: some central issues. *Journal of Adolescence, 20*, 333–342.

Fung, K.M.T., Tsang, H.W.H., Corrigan, P.W., Lam, C.S., & Cheung, W.M. (2007). Measuring self-stigma of mental illness in China and its implications for recovery. *International Journal of Social Psychiatry, 53*, 408–418.

Goffman, E. (1963). *Stigma: Notes on the Management of Spoiled Identity*. Englewood Cliffs, NJ: Prentice-Hall.

Hammarstroem, A., & Janlert, U. (1997). Nervous and depressive symptoms in a longitudinal study of youth unemployment: selection or exposure? *Journal of Adolescence, 20*, 293–305.

Hand, C., & Tryssenaar, J. (2006). Small business employers' views on hiring individuals with mental illness. *Psychiatric Rehabilitation Journal, 29*, 166–173.

Hatfield, B., Huxley, P., & Mohamad, H. (1992). Accommodation and employment: a survey into the circumstances and expressed needs of users of mental health services in a northern town. *British Journal of Social Work, 22*, 61–73.

Henry, A.D., & Lucca, A.M. (2004). Facilitators and barriers to employment: the perspectives of people with psychiatric disabilities and employment service providers. *Work, 22*, 169–182.

Holmes, E.P., Corrigan, P.W., Williams, P., Canar, J., & Kubiak, M.A. (1999). Changing public attitudes about schizophrenia. *Schizophrenia Bulletin, 25*, 447–456.

Johnson, V.A., Greenwood, R., & Schriner, K.F. (1988). Work performance and work personality: employer concerns about workers with disabilities. *Rehabilitation Counseling Bulletin, 32*, 50–57.

Johnson-Dalzine, P., Dalzine, L., & Martin-Stanley, C. (1996). Fear of criminal violence and the African American elderly: assessment of a crime prevention strategy. *Journal of Negro Education, 65*, 462–469.

Jorm, A.F. (2000). Mental health literacy: public knowledge and beliefs about mental disorders. *British Journal of Psychiatry, 177*, 396–401.

Jorm, A.F., Korten, A.E., Jacomb, P.A., Christensen, H., Rodgers, B., & Pollitt, P. (1997). "Mental health literacy": a survey of the public's ability to recognise mental disorders and their beliefs about the effectiveness of treatment. *Medical Journal of Australia, 166*, 182–186.

Keane, M.C. (1991). Acceptance vs. rejection: nursing students' attitudes about mental illness. *Perspectives in Psychiatric Care, 27*, 13–18.

King, A.Y.C., & Bond, M.H. (1985). The Confucian paradigm of man: a sociological view. In: Tseng, W.S., & Wu, D.Y.H. (eds). *Chinese Culture and Mental Health*. Orlando, FL: Academic Press, pp. 29–45.

Link, B.G. (1982). Mental patient status, work, and income: an examination of the effects of a psychiatric label. *American Sociological Review, 47*, 202–215.

Link, B.G. (1987). Understanding labeling effects in the area of mental disorders: an assessment of the effects of expectations of rejection. *American Sociological Review*, 52, 96–112.

Link, B.G., & Cullen, F.T. (1986). Contact with the mentally ill and perceptions of how dangerous they are. *Journal of Health and Social Behavior*, 27, 289–302.

Link, B.G., Cullen, F.T., Frank, J., & Wozniak, J.F. (1987). The social rejection of former mental patients: understanding why labels matter. *American Journal of Sociology*, 92, 1461–1500.

Link, B.G., Phelan, J.C., Bresnahan, M., Stueve, A., & Pescosolido, B.A. (1999). Public conceptions of mental illness: labels, causes, dangerousness, and social distance. *American Journal of Public Health*, 89, 1328–1333.

Macrae, C., Bodenhausen, G.V., Milne, A.B., & Jetten, J. (1994). Out of mind but back in sight: stereotypes on the rebound. *Journal of Personality and Social Psychology*, 67, 808–817.

Mak, C.S., Tsang, H.W.H., & Cheung, L.C.C. (2006). Job termination among individuals with severe mental illness participated in a supported employment program in Hong Kong. *Psychiatry*, 69, 239–248.

Manning, C., & White, P.D. (1995). Attitudes of employers to the mentally ill. *Psychiatric Bulletin*, 19, 541–543.

Marwaha, S., & Johnson, S. (2004). Schizophrenia and employment. *Social Psychiatry and Psychiatric Epidemiology*, 39, 337–349.

Morgan, G. (2005). We want to be able to work. *Mental Health Today October*, 32–34.

Morrison, J.K. (1980). The public's current beliefs about mental illness: serious obstacle to effective community psychology. *American Journal of Community Psychology*, 8, 697–707.

Morrison, J.K., Cocozza, J.J., & Vanderwyst, D. (1980). An attempt to change the negative, stigmatizing image of mental patients through brief reeducation. *Psychological Reports*, 47, 334.

Morrison, J.K., & Teta, D.C. (1980). Reducing students' fear of mental illness by means of seminar-induced belief change. *Journal of Clinical Psychology*, 36, 275–276.

Olshanksy, S., Grob, S., & Ekdahl, M. (1960). Survey of employment experience of patients discharged from three mental hospitals during the period 1951–1953. *Mental Hygiene*, 44, 510–521.

Pearson, V. (1995). *Mental Health Care in China: State Policies, Professional Services and Family Responsibilities*. London: Gaskell.

Penn, D.L., Guynan, K., Daily, T., Spaulding, W.D., Garbin, C.P., & Sullivan, M. (1994). Dispelling the stigma of schizophrenia: what sort of information is best? *Schizophrenia Bulletin*, 20, 567–578.

Penn, D.L., Kommana, S., Mansfield, M., & Link, B.G. (1999). Dispelling the stigma of schizophrenia. II: The impact of information on dangerousness. *Schizophrenia Bulletin*, 25, 437–446.

Pescosolido, B.A., Monahan, J., Link, B.G., Stueve, A., & Kikuzawa, S. (1999). The public's view of the competence, dangerousness, and need for legal coercion of persons with mental health problems. *American Journal of Public Health*, 89, 1339–1345.

Peterson, D., Pere, L., Sheehan, N., & Surgenor, G. (2006). Experience of mental health discrimination in New Zealand. *Health and Social Care in the Community*, 15, 18–25.

Rinaldi, M., & Hill, R. (2000). *Insufficient Concern*. London: Merton Mind.

Ritsher, J.B., & Phelan, J.C. (2004). Internalized stigma predicts erosion of morale among psychiatric outpatients. *Psychiatric Research*, 129, 257–265.

Rochlin, J. (1987). Rehabilitation: an employer's perspective. *Rehabilitation Education*, *1*, 89–94.

Roman, P., & Floyd, H.H. (1981). Social acceptance of psychiatric illness and psychiatric treatment. *Social Psychiatry*, *16*, 16–21.

Rosenheck, R.A., Leslie, D., Keefe, R., McEvoy, J., Swartz, M., Perkins, D., Stroup, S., Hsiao, J.K., Liberman, J., & the CATIE Study Investigation Group (2006). Barriers to employment for people with schizophrenia. *American Journal of Psychiatry*, *163*, 411–417.

Rusch, N., Angermeyer, M.C., & Corrigan, P.W. (2005). Mental illness stigma: concepts, consequences, and initiatives to reduce stigma. *European Psychiatry*, *20*, 529–539.

Sainfort, F., Becker, M., & Diamond, R. (1996). Judgements of quality of life of individuals with severe mental disorders: patients' self-report vs. providers' perspectives. *American Journal of Psychiatry*, *4*, 497–502.

Schaufeli, W.B. (1997). Youth unemployment and mental health: some Dutch findings. *Journal of Adolescence*, *20*, 281–292.

Scheid, T.L. (2005). Stigma as a barrier to employment: mental disability and the Americans with Disabilities Act. *International Journal of Law and Psychiatry*, *28*, 670–690.

Schulze, B., & Angermeyer, M.C. (2003). Subjective experience of stigma: a focus group study of schizophrenic patients, their relatives and mental health professionals. *Social Science & Medicine*, *56*, 299–312.

Schumacher, M., Corrigan, P.W., & Dejong, T. (2003). Examining cues that signal mental illness stigma. *Journal of Social and Clinical Psychology*, *22*, 467–476.

Secker, J., Grove, B., & Seebohm, P. (2001). Challenging barriers to employment, training and education for mental health service users: the service user's perspective. *Journal of Mental Health*, *10*, 395–404.

Siu, P.S.K., Tsang, H.W.H., & Bond, G.R. (in press). Nonvocational outcomes for clients with severe mental illness obtaining employment in Hong Kong. *Community Mental Health Journal*.

South Essex Service User Research Group, Secker, J., & Gelling, L. (2006). Still dreaming: service users' employment, education and training goals. *Journal of Mental Health*, *15*, 103–111.

Stuart, H. (2006). Employment equity and mental disability. *Current Opinion Psychiatry*, *20*, 486–490.

Surgeon General. (2000). *Mental Health: A Report of the Surgeon General*. Rockville, MD: U.S. Public Health Office.

Tanaka, G., Ogawa, T., Inadomi, H., Kikuchi, Y., & Ohta, Y. (2003). Effects of an educational program on public attitudes towards mental illness. *Psychiatry and Clinical Neurosciences*, *57*, 595–602.

Taylor, S.M., & Dear, M.J. (1981). Scaling community attitudes toward the mentally-ill. *Schizophrenia Bulletin*, *7*, 225–240.

Thomas, T.D., Thomas, G., & Joiner, J.G. (1993). Issues in the vocational rehabilitation of persons with serious and persistent mental illness: a national survey of counselor insights. *Psychosocial Rehabilitation Journal*, *16*, 129–134.

Thornton, J.A., & Wahl, O.F. (1996). Impact of a newspaper article on attitudes towards mental illness. *Journal of Community Psychology*, *24*, 17–25.

Tsang, H.W.H. (2003). Augmenting vocational outcomes of supported employment by social skills training. *Journal of Rehabilitation*, *69*, 25–30.

Tsang, H.W.H., Angell, B., Corrigan, P.W., Lee, Y.T., Shi, K., Lam, C.S., Jin, S., & Fung, K.M.T. (2007). A cross-cultural study of employers' concerns about hiring people with psychotic disorder: implications for recovery. *Social Psychiatry and Psychiatric Epidemiology*, 42, 723–733.

Tsang, H.W.H., Chan, A., Wong, A., & Liberman, R.P. (2009). Vocational outcomes of an integrated supported employment program for individuals with persistent and severe mental illness. *Journal of Behavior Therapy and Experimental Psychiatry*, 40(2), 292–305.

Tsang, H.W.H., & Pearson, V. (2001). A work-related social skills training for people with schizophrenia in Hong Kong. *Schizophrenia Bulletin*, 27, 139–148.

Tsang, H.W.H., Tam, P., Chan, F., & Cheung, W.M. (2003). Stigmatizing attitudes towards individuals with mental illness in Hong Kong: implications to their recovery. *Journal of Community Psychology*, 31, 383–396.

Tu, W.M. (1998). Confucius and Confucianism. In Slote, W.H., & DeVos, G.A. (eds), *Confucianism and the Family*. Albany, NY: State University of New York Press, pp. 3–36.

Vauth, R., Kleim, B., Wirtz, M., & Corrigan, P.W. (2007). Self-efficacy and empowerment as outcomes of self-stigmatizing and coping in schizophrenia. *Psychiatry Research*, 150, 71–80.

Wahl, O.F. (1995). *Media Madness: Public Images of Mental Illness*. New Brunswick, NJ: Rutgers University Press.

Wahl, O.F. (1999). Mental health consumers' experience of stigma. *Schizophrenia Bulletin*, 25, 467–478.

Warr, P.B., Jackson, P., & Banks, M. (1988). Unemployment and mental health: some British studies. *Journal of Social Issues*, 44, 47–68.

Webber, A., & Orcutt, J. (1984). Employers' reactions to racial and psychiatric stigma: a field experiment. *Deviant Behavior*, 5, 327–336.

Wilgosh, L., & Skaret, D. (1987). Employer attitudes toward hiring individuals with disabilities: a review of the recent literature. *Canadian Journal of Rehabilitation*, 1, 89–98.

Wong, K.K., Chiu, R., Tang, B., Chiu, S.N., & Tang, J.L. (2006). *Hong Kong: Health Services Research Committee Dissemination Report: A Randomized Controlled Trial of a Supported Employment Program on Vocational Outcomes of Individuals with Chronic Mental Illness*. Hong Kong: The Hong Kong Polytechnic University.

Yao, X. (2000). *An Introduction to Confucianism*. Cambridge, UK: Cambridge University Press.

Yip, K.S. (2005). Coping with public labeling of clients with mental illness in Hong Kong: a report of personal experiences. *International Journal of Psychosocial Rehabilitation*, 9, 1–15.

Chapter 5
MOTIVATIONAL INTERVIEWING

Chris Lloyd and Robert King

Chapter overview

People with mental illness are overrepresented among those who are not seeking employment assistance and those not actively looking for work, and are underrepresented among those currently employed. Motivational barriers prevent many from attempting to enter the workforce or to seek help from the specialist services available. We suggest that clinicians consider motivational interviewing as a means of assisting clients clarify and enhance motivation for change and resolve ambivalence about employment. Previous research supports the use of motivational interviewing for assisting people with mental illness with a variety of life problems. This chapter describes motivational interviewing, highlights some of the previous research and looks at its application in relation to employment for people with a mental illness.

Introduction

This chapter will examine:

- Motivational interviewing
- Previous research
- Employment and barriers to employment
- Motivational interviewing and employment

Motivational interviewing

Spirit of motivational interviewing

One of the key components of the spirit of motivational interviewing is its collaborative nature. Counselling involves a partnership with the client and focuses on exploration and support. The interviewer seeks to create a positive interpersonal atmosphere that is conducive to change (Miller & Rollnick, 2002). Consistent with a collaborative role, the interviewer's position is one of enquiry with the aim of understanding (and helping the client to understand) internal motivational struggles. Responsibility for change is left with the client. Respect is shown for the client's autonomy. The overall goal is to enable the client to become clearer about intrinsic motivation, so that the change arises from within rather than being imposed upon the person, therefore serving the person's own goals and values (Miller & Rollnick, 2002).

The transtheoretical model of change

Motivational interviewing takes place within a broad framework termed the Transtheoretical Model of Change, more commonly known as the Stages of Change Model (Prochaska et al., 1992). According to this model, the process of change requires that individuals move through a series of stages from precontemplation to maintenance. Following are brief descriptions of each of these four stages. They are accompanied by sample items from a widely used questionnaire designed to evaluate a person's stage of change. The University of Rhode Island Change Assessment Scale (URICA) was developed to measure the stages of change (McConnaughy et al., 1983). It operationally defines four theoretical stages of change: Precontemplation, Contemplation, Action and Maintenance. The scale consists of 32 items, with eight items measuring each of the change subscales. Responses are given on a five-point Likert format (1= strong disagreement to 5 = strong agreement).

Precontemplation

Precontemplation is the stage at which there is no intention to change behaviour in the foreseeable future. Items that are used to identify precontemplation include 'As far as I' concerned, I don't have any problems that need changing' and ' I guess I have faults, but there is nothing that I really need to change'. Resistance to recognising or modifying is the key issue in precontemplation (Prochaska et al., 1992). There may be recognition that others perceive a need for change but no overt acknowledgement of internal motivation for change.

Contemplation

Contemplation is the stage when people are aware that a problem exists but have not yet made a commitment to action. Items used to measure contemplators include 'I have a problem and I really think I should work on it' and 'I've been thinking that I might want to change something about myself'. In the contemplation phase there is often a wish for change but no belief in the capacity to change (no self-efficacy).

Action

Action is the stage in which individuals modify their behaviour, experiences or environment in order to overcome their problem. Items include 'I am really working hard to change' and 'Anyone can talk about changing, I am actually doing something about it'.

Maintenance

Maintenance is the stage in which people work to prevent relapse and consolidate the changes made during the action stage. Maintenance items include 'I may need a boost right now to help me maintain the changes I've already made' and 'I'm here to prevent myself from having a relapse of my problem'.

Relapse and recycling through the stages occur quite frequently as people attempt to modify or change their behaviours. Prochaska et al. (1992) proposed a spiral pattern of how most people actually move through the stages of change. In this spiral pattern, people can progress from contemplation to preparation to action to maintenance, but most people will relapse. During relapse, people will regress to an earlier stage. They suggested that each time relapsers recycle through the stages they potentially learn from their mistakes and can try something different the next time around.

Motivational interviewing and stages of change

The general strategy of motivational interviewing is to help people progress from one stage to the next. As the issues and interviewing strategies will change according to the stages, it is important that the clinician has a good sense of the stage a client is at each interview. Because slippage can easily occur in the course of change, it is unwise to make assumptions about the stage of change even when the therapeutic work is ongoing.

Four general principles of motivational interviewing

Four broad guiding principles underlie motivational interviewing as a clinical technique. These principles are express empathy, develop discrepancy, roll with resistance and support self-efficacy.

Express empathy

Through skilful reflective listening, the therapist seeks to understand the client's feelings and perspectives without judging, criticising or blaming. It is possible to accept and understand the person's perspective while not agreeing with or endorsing it. Reluctance to change problematic behaviour is to be expected in treatment settings (Miller & Rollnick, 2002). Although clinicians are taught reflective, non-judgemental listening, many find this counter-intuitive when the client is saying things the clinician does not agree with or does not want to hear. For example, clinicians often do find it difficult to express empathy when a client indicates he enjoys cannabis and just 'hanging out'. However, it is an essential requirement of motivational interviewing that the clinician engage in empathic reflective listening so that both the clinician and the client get a better understanding of what makes this kind of activity enjoyable and how it impacts on other goals and motivations. Unless both client and clinician have the full picture, decisions that lead to change are unlikely to occur. This means the clinician has to control the impulse to either challenge the client or change the topic and instead be willing to enter into the client's motivational world.

Develop discrepancy

The decisions people make result from complex psychological forces and are partly influenced by core values and long-term goals and partly by short-term considerations such as immediate gratification or avoidance of discomfort. This means that people are often conflicted – achieving a long-term goal may mean having to cope with short-term discomfort. Because most people dislike psychological conflict, we tend to resolve the conflict by banishing part of the conflict from conscious awareness. In other words, if I want to avoid immediate discomfort but know that it will cost in relation to long-term goals, a solution is to pretend that I do not have any long-term goals. Motivational interviewing aims to reintroduce the conflict. This means assisting the client to recognise a discrepancy between present behaviour and his or her broader goals and values. This often means an approach to enquiry designed to elicit core values and long-term goals. The motivational interviewing process helps the client to recognise a discrepancy between current behaviour and core values and long-term goals. Once this discrepancy is activated, the client has to resolve the internal conflict and this may mean change in current patterns of behaviour (Miller & Rollnick, 2002). The key to successful motivational interviewing is that the client is the person who recognises and deals with the discrepancy. It is not the job of the interviewer to point out the discrepancy, but rather to elicit values and goals and then invite the client to consider both current behaviour and core values and long-term goals.

Roll with resistance

One strategy that people often use to deal with discrepancy is to externalise part of the internal conflict. What this means is that the person takes the position that the goals are not theirs but those of the interviewer. The more a person can get into an argument with someone else, the less they have to deal with internal conflict. Therapists and counsellors can easily find themselves getting into some kind of argument in which they are pushing for a change and the client is resisting. In motivational interviewing, we want the argument to be an internal one for the client. This means that the practitioner does not impose new views or goals. Instead, the person is invited to consider the new information and is offered new perspectives. As soon as the practitioner notices resistance she or he backs off, making it clear that any decisions or choices are for the client to make. Rolling with resistance means that the therapist does become an active player in the argument and the client is at the centre of the process of problem solving (Miller & Rollnick, 2002).

Support self-efficacy

Self-efficacy refers to a person's belief in his or her ability to carry out and succeed with a specific task. It is a key element in the transition from a wish for change to change in behaviour (in change jargon, from contemplation to action). A general goal of motivational interviewing is to enhance a client's confidence in his or her capability to cope with obstacles and to succeed in change (Miller & Rollnick, 2002). This means sensitivity to what the client actually feels capable of doing. Therapists have to be careful not to push clients beyond their self-efficacy and not to take steps on behalf of the client because the client does not yet feel ready to take those steps.

Evaluating motivation and self-efficacy

At various points in the motivational interviewing process, it is useful to get a quantitative indication of the strength of motivation for change and the strength of self-efficacy with respect to the changes in behaviour that would be required to achieve changes. Miller and Rollnick (2002) recommend the use of a simple scale with gradations from 0 to 10 to evaluate these two dimensions (Box 5.1).

The idea is to end up knowing how important the client perceives change to be and how confident the person is that he or she could do it.

Setting the scene

The very first session can be crucial as it sets both the tone and the expectations for therapy. A good structuring statement can set the client's mind at rest and get the intervention off to a good start. Miller and Rollnick (2002, p. 64) suggest that the following elements could be included:

- The amount of time you have available
- An explanation of your role and goals

Box 5.1 Importance and confidence.

How important would you say it is for you to_____? On a scale from 0 to 10, where 0 is 'not at all important' and 10 is 'extremely important'. Where would you say you are?

0	1	2	3	4	5	6	7	8	9	10

Not at all important   Extremely important

And how confident would you say you are, that if you decided to_____, you could do it? On the same scale from 0 to 10, where 0 is 'not at all confident' and 10 is 'extremely confident', where would you say you are?

- A description of the client's role
- A mention of details that must be attended to
- An open-ended question

Agenda setting is important so a basic question of 'what are you going to talk about' is useful.

Early methods

They are called 'early' methods because it is important to be using them right from the start. The first four methods are summarised by the acronym OARS (open questions, affirming, reflecting and summarising). These techniques are very similar to active listening techniques that have long been central to non-directive counselling.

In the interview situation, the client should do most of the talking, with the practitioner listening carefully and encouraging expression. One key for encouraging clients do most of the talking is to ask open questions, i.e. questions that do not invite brief answers. The general pattern in motivational interviewing is to ask an open question, set the topic of exploration and then follow with reflective listening (Miller & Rollnick, 2002).

Directly affirming and supporting the client during the counselling process is another way of building rapport and reinforcing open exploration. It is important to notice and appropriately affirm the client's strengths and efforts (Miller & Rollnick, 2002).

Reflective listening is one of the most important and most challenging skills required for motivational interviewing. Reflective listening is feedback to the client that shows you understand what the client is communicating. It may focus on content (cognitive dimension) or emotion (affective dimension) or both. It often involves a paraphrase rather than a simple claim to understand.

If the therapist simply says 'I see what you mean' then the client does not know whether the therapist really understands or is just saying he or she understands. On the other hand, 'sounds like you find it really disheartening when people tell you to just stop smoking' indicates that you have understood both the content and the emotion. It is often useful to understate slightly what the speaker has offered (Miller & Rollnick, 2002).

The fourth OARS method to use early and throughout motivational interviewing is summarising. Summary statements can be used to link together and reinforce material that has been discussed. It is a good idea to summarise periodically since they reinforce what has been said, show that the practitioner has been listening carefully and prepare the client to elaborate further (Miller & Rollnick, 2002). An example of a summary might be 'What I have heard you say so far is you would really like to get a job because it would be good to have some extra money and you know it would really please your parents, but you worry that you won't be able to work properly because you have problems with concentration and you also worry that stress from working could make your mental illness worse'.

Methods for evoking change talk

Evoking change talk is one of the key motivational interviewing skills. Open-ended questions can be used to explore the client's own perceptions and concerns. The scale described above can be used to obtain the client's own rating of importance. Miller and Rollnick (2002) suggest that two questions are asked: 'Why are at a _____ and not zero?' and 'What would it take for you to go from _____ to [a higher number]?'

Decisional balance

Once it is established that the client is at least willing to contemplate change, it is important for both the client and the therapist to clarify the internal conflicts that are relevant to a decision – whether that be a decision to change or a decision not to change. This is determined decisional balance, and an effective technique to clarify decisional balance is to encourage the client to draw up a balance sheet listing the pros and cons for change. This is best done in a collaborative manner using a whiteboard or a large sheet of paper thatboth the client and the therapist can see.

The example below is with a client who has a mental illness and is contemplating moving towards employment. The person is in receipt of a social security benefit (Box 5.2).

When all the decisional considerations have been identified, it is up to the client to weigh them up and think about what they mean in terms of behaviour challenge. The therapist has to resist the temptation to actively step-in to tip

---

Box 5.2   A decisional balance sheet.

Continue to be unemployed	Seek employment/start work
No responsibility – I might let people down if I was working	More money – it would be great to be able to afford a decent sound system
Can sleep in – nice not having a routine	Family will be proud of me
Low stress – I would worry about failing and about what people think of me (especially if they know I have a mental illness) if I was working	Start to a long-term future – I have always wanted to have a career and be able to buy a house
No risk to social security payments – I have a disability support pension and they can take it of you if you are working.	Better chance of getting a girlfriend – I get lonely on my own and sometimes I even think it would be nice to have a kiss

---

the balance but it is OK to remind the client about core values and long-term goals and to ask how a decision, one way or the other, would impact on these.

If the client indicates a wish for behaviour change, this is only the first step. This wish has to become a commitment and then a realistic prospect. The next step is to move towards commitment, and according to Miller and Rollnick (2002, p. 80), a useful step is to elicit elaboration once a reason for change has been raised. This might involve:

- Asking for clarification: In what ways? How much? When?
- Asking for a specific example
- Asking for a description of the last time this occurred
- Asking 'What else?' within the change topic

When there appears to be little desire for change at present, another way to elicit change talk is to ask people to describe the extremes of their concerns and to imagine the extreme consequences that might take place. Sometimes it is useful when eliciting change talk to have the client remember times before the problem emerged and to compare those times with the present situation. Helping people envision a changed future is another approach for eliciting change talk. Returning to core values – what things are the most important in his or her life – is helpful in this respect. When the client's highest goals are defined, the practitioner can ask how the problem that has been discussed fits into this picture (Miller & Rollnick, 2002).

Negotiating a change plan

The development of a change plan is a process of shared decision-making and negotiation that involves:

- Setting goals
- Considering change options
- Arriving at a plan
- Developing commitment to the plan
- Developing self-efficacy in relation to the steps required to execute the plan (Miller & Rollnick, 2002, p. 133)

A first step in instigating change is to have a goal to work towards. The practitioner can ask for a confidence rating and ask the client to consider what consequences may follow from taking this particular course of action. It is a good idea to prioritise goals through a process of shared decision-making. If the client is expressing doubts about a goal, there is more work to do before proceeding (Miller & Rollnick, 2002).

Once the person's goal has been clarified, the next step is to consider possible methods or means for achieving the chosen goal. Involve the client in brain-storming and evaluating possible change strategies. A key focus is to draw on a person's own internal resources and natural social support (Miller & Rollnick, 2002).

Elicit the change plan by having the client voice it. It may be useful to fill in a written change plan, summarizing what it is that the client plans to do (Box 5.3).

Box 5.3   A change plan worksheet.

The most important reasons why I want to make this change are:

My main goals for myself in making this change are:

I plan to do these things in order to accomplish my goals:

Specific action	When

Other people could help me with change in these ways

Person:	Possible ways to help

These are some possible obstacles to change, and how I could handle them

Possible obstacles to change	How to respond

I will know that my plan is working when I see these results

A change plan is a strategy for change. It provides a reference point and a guide but it should always be open to revision if parts are not working in practice. It can sometimes be helpful for the client to make the plan public. The client can visit or telephone other people to let them know about the plan and to ask for their help. The commitment to a change plan completes the formal cycle of motivational interviewing (Miller & Rollnick, 2002).

The effectiveness of motivational interviewing: research findings

Motivational interviewing has been extensively researched with a wide range of clients and problems. Several studies have undertaken a systematic review or meta-analysis to summarise findings from multiple individual studies.

Rubak et al. (2005) undertook a systematic review and meta-analysis of randomised controlled trials using motivational interviewing as the intervention. They found that motivational interviewing in a scientific setting outperforms traditional advice given in the treatment of a broad range of behavioural problems and diseases. Dunn et al. (2001) conducted a systematic review to examine the effectiveness of brief behavioural interventions adapting the principles and techniques of motivational interviewing. There was substantial evidence that motivational interviewing is an effective substance abuse intervention method, particularly as an enhancement to more intensive treatment. Burke et al. (2003) conducted a meta-analysis on controlled clinical trials investigating adaptations of motivational interviewing. Results indicated that the motivational interviewing-based intervention was equivalent to other active treatments and yielded moderate effects compared with no treatment for problems involving alcohol, drugs, diet and exercise. Britt et al. (2004) conducted a review of the use of motivational interviewing in health care settings. They concluded that motivational interviewing appears to hold substantial promise for health behaviour change as it is consistent with the call for a more client-centred approach in health care in which the health practitioner–client relationship is seen as a partnership rather than an expert-recipient one. They further concluded that motivational interviewing provides health practitioners with a means of tailoring their interventions to suit the client's degree of readiness to change and with an effective means of working with clients who are ambivalent about, or not ready for, change. Chanut et al. (2005) reviewed studies investigating motivational interviewing with people with mental health problems and found generally shown positive results, especially increased engagement and adherence. They concluded from the literature that significant change can occur quite rapidly with this population.

In summary, while motivational interviewing is not a panacea and clinicians cannot be assured of positive results, there is now a large body of work affirming its value. Of particular relevance to this chapter is evidence of its applicability to people affected by mental illness.

Employment

Working is a core part of modern life, providing an opportunity to participate fully in the society (Marwaha et al., 2008). Employment provides social contacts and social support, status and identity, a means of structuring and occupying time and a sense of personal achievement (Perkins & Rinaldi, 2002). Despite high unemployment rates, people with mental illness report the desire to work and view employment as an important recovery goal (McQuilken et al., 2003; Provencher et al., 2002). If the majority of people with mental illness want to work, why are so few actually working? Research indicates that there are a variety of reasons, including financial disincentives – the effect on their disability pensions (McQuilken et al., 2003), stigma and employment discrimination (Rosenheck et al., 2006), illness-related problems (Johannensen et al., 2007; Rosenheck et al., 2006) and poor illness management (Tschopp et al., 2007), low expectations of staff and negative staff attitudes (Marwaha et al., 2008), past difficulty in keeping a job and low self-confidence (Johannensen et al., 2007) and environmental factors such as transportation problems (Johannensen et al., 2007).

People with mental illness often require assistance to overcome these barriers. Fortunately there are well-established programmes with a track record for success in facilitating entry into the workforce for people with severe mental illness. Supported employment programmes such as Individual Placement and Support have the overriding philosophy that anyone is capable of working competitively in the community if the right kind of job and work environment can be found and the right kind of support is provided (Rinaldi et al., 2008). Supported employment programmes provide work opportunities for people with mental illness who might otherwise have difficulty securing integrated and competitive employment (Tschopp et al., 2007). Clubhouses also have a successful track record in facilitating access to work through transitional and supported employment (Schonebaum et al., 2006) and, in addition, provide members with a supportive and collegial peer network.

Overcoming barriers to employment is a major motivational challenge, and it is not surprising that people with severe mental illness often decide not to attempt to enter the workforce. For many, even seeking help is a motivational challenge. However, it is evident that for many, there will be substantial ambivalence in relation to decisions regarding employment. One part of the person, often the part associated with core values and long-term goals will see work as being attractive and desirable. Another part of the person will feel highly apprehensive about the possible adverse consequences of seeking work and will find the prospect of working quite unattractive. For this reason, issues around employment and seeking help to access employment are well suited to the motivational interviewing approach discussed above.

Although the use of motivational interviewing to assist people to resolve motivational conflicts associated with employment has not been extensively studied, there is already some evidence that it is likely to be helpful. Larson et al. (2007) introduced motivational interviewing into an Individual Placement and Support-supported employment and found that programme participants significantly increased the number of obtained jobs, hours worked per week, hourly wage and monthly job income. Participants' stage of change was found to be positively correlated with jobs offered, jobs obtained and hourly wage.

Graham et al. (2008) looked at the potential for the techniques within motivational interviewing to add value to employment assessments. They proposed that motivational interviewing be used as a technique that would allow practitioners to involve clients in resolving their ambivalence about work and employment opportunities. It was suggested that these techniques would provide practitioners with the tools to strengthen the level of commitment and engagement of previously resistant clients in activities that would help them make progress towards work. Likewise, Lloyd et al. (2008) proposed using motivational interviewing to assist people with mental illness to clarify their motivation for work. They suggested that motivational interviewing be used to assist people with mental illness form vocational goals.

Conclusions

Motivational interviewing takes the position that all behaviour involves decisions – even when we are not aware of them. Not changing involves a decision. Motivational interviewing is an approach to counselling designed to assist people to make better decisions about behaviour change. It does this by supporting the person to recognise rather than avoid ambivalence and to take into account core values and long-term goals when making decisions. It employs widely used counselling techniques such as active listening, but also requires clinicians to understand and respect motivations they may not agree with – which can be challenging and counter-intuitive. Motivational interviewing has been extensively researched and has consistently been found to assist with decision-making and behaviour change. For people affected by severe mental illness, decisions to seek employment are difficult because, while working may be consistent with core values and long-term goals, there are many obstacles and barriers to be overcome. Research so far suggests that motivational interviewing may provide clinicians with an effective strategy for assisting clients to work their way through the motivational challenges associated with employment.

References

Britt, E., Hudson, S.M., & Blampied, N.M. (2004). Motivational interviewing in health care: a review. *Patient Educational and Counseling*, *53*, 147–155.

Burke, B.L., Arkowitz, H., & Menchola, M. (2003). The efficacy of motivational interviewing: a meta-analysis of controlled clinical trials. *Journal of Consulting and Clinical Psychology*, *71*, 843–861.

Chanut, F., Brown, T.G., & Dongier, M. (2005). Motivational interviewing and clinical psychiatry. *Canadian Journal of Psychiatry*, *50*, 715–721.

Dunn, C., Deroo, L., & Rivara, F.P. (2001). The use of brief interventions adapted from motivational interviewing across behavioral domains: a systematic review. *Addiction*, *96*, 1725–1742.

Graham, V., Jutla, S., Higginson, D., & Wells, A. (2008). The added value of Motivational Interviewing within employment assessments. *Journal of Occupational Psychology, Employment and Disability*, *10*, 43–52.

Johannensen, J.K., McGrew, J.H., Griss, M.E., & Born, D. (2007). Perception of illness as a barrier to work in consumers of supported employment programs. *Journal of Vocational Rehabilitation*, *27*, 39–47.

Larson, J.E., Barr, L.K., Boyle, M.G., & Glenn, T.L. (2007). Process and outcome analysis of a supported employment program for people with psychiatric disabilities. *American Journal of Psychiatric Rehabilitation*, *10*, 339–353.

Lloyd, C., Tse, S., Waghorn, G., & Hennessy, N. (2008). Motivational interviewing in vocational rehabilitation for people living with mental ill health. *International Journal of Therapy and Rehabilitation*, *15*, 572–579.

Marwaha, S., Balachandra, S., & Johnson, S. (2008). Clinicians' attitude to the employment of people with psychosis. *Social Psychiatry and Psychiatric Epidemiology*, *44*, 349–360.

McConnaughy, E.A., Prochaska, J.O., & Velicer, W.F. (1983). Stages of change in psychotherapy: measurement and sample profiles. *Psychotherapy: Theory, Research and Practice*, *20*, 368–375.

McQuilken, M., Zahniser, J.H., Novak, J., Starks, R.D., Olmos, A., & Bond, G.R. (2003). The work project survey: consumer perspectives on work. *Journal of Vocational Rehabilitation*, *18*, 59–68.

Miller, W.R., & Rollnick, S. (2002). *Motivational Interviewing – Preparing People for Change*, 2nd edn. New York: The Guildford Press.

Perkins, R., & Rinaldi, M. (2002). Unemployment among patients with long-term mental health problems. *Psychiatric Bulletin*, *26*, 295–298.

Prochaska, J.O., DeClemente, C.C., & Norcross, J.C. (1992). In search of how people change – applications to addictive behaviors. *American Psychologist*, *42*(9), 1102–1114.

Provencher, H.L., Gregg, R., Mead, S, & Mueser, K.T. (2002). The role of work in the recovery of persons with psychiatric disabilities. *Psychiatric Rehabilitation Journal*, *26*, 132–146.

Rinaldi, M., Perkins, R., Glynn, E., Montibeller, T., Clenaghan, M., & Rutherford, J. (2008). Individual placement and support: from research to practice. *Advances in Psychiatric Treatment*, *14*, 50–60.

Rosenheck, R., Leslie, D., Keefe, R., McEvoy, J., Swartz, M., Perkins, D., Stroup, S., Hsiao, J.K., & Liberman, J. (2006). Barriers to employment for people with schizophrenia. *American Journal of Psychiatry*, *163*, 411–417.

Rubak, S., Sandbaek, A., Laluritzen, T., & Christensen, B. (2005). Motivational interviewing: a systematic review and meta-analysis. *British Journal of General Practice*, *55*, 305–312.

Schonebaum, A., Boyd J., & Dudek K. (2006). A comparison of competitive employment outcomes for the clubhouse and PACT models. *Psychiatric Services*, *57*, 1416–1420.

Tschopp, M.K., Perkins, D.V., Hart-Katuin, C., Born, D.L., & Holt, S.L. (2007). Employment barriers and strategies for individuals with psychiatric disabilities and criminal histories. *Journal of Vocational Rehabilitation*, *26*, 175–187.

Chapter 6

WHEN MOTIVATION FOR VOCATIONAL ASSISTANCE IS UNCLEAR

Terry Krupa

Chapter overview

Despite advancements in the development of vocational services which improve employment outcomes, there has been a lack of direct attention to problems related to motivation for employment which are experienced by people with mental illness. Addressing these motivational problems will require a comprehensive understanding of underlying personal, environmental and occupational factors. Personal factors include issues related to self-efficacy and the capacity for pleasurable affective experiences and emotional rewards associated with employment. Environmental factors include social stigma that is internalised by the individual, constraints related to finances and poverty, and formal and informal social supports that have the power to enable or undermine employment motivation. Occupation factors relate to the personal and social meaning inherent in work. Contemporary evidence-based approaches to employment support integrate principled practices that can facilitate motivation for employment. In addition, vocational service providers can work collaboratively with individuals to use targeted strategies to address motivational problems, including motivational interviewing, standardised assessments and collaborative psychopharmacology; eliciting the power of affective and emotional rewards of work; cognitive-behavioural therapy, peer support, disclosure counselling and benefits counselling.

Introduction

Dion has been meeting with a mental health vocational specialist to develop employment plans. The vocational service matches people with mental illness with the jobs they want and then provides the support they require to be successful in these jobs. Dion is 23 years old. About a year ago he was working as an assistant in a laboratory following an unsuccessful attempt at university-level studies in science. He quit his job when he was hospitalised with his first episode of psychosis. Now that he is recovering from his experience of mental illness he would like to get on with his life, and in particular employment. He appreciates the help he is receiving in finding work but at the same time he finds that he is troubled by feelings of ambivalence about following through with employment plans. He describes himself as having a 'lack of purpose and direction', a disquieting feeling of 'lack of enthusiasm' and an overall sense of 'discomfort with himself'. He simultaneously wants to work in the community and to withdraw from social contacts and responsibilities. The information he has received about the mental illness has him worried that things 'might not get much better'.

The concerns that Dion is experiencing are fairly common among people with mental illness who are engaging with vocational services with a view to returning to employment. Dion demonstrates how an individual can have a genuine desire for employment and yet be weighed down by uncertainty and uneasiness that have the potential to undermine focused efforts towards employment. The case highlights that vocational service providers need to be prepared to address motivational issues that can compromise employment. Vocational services that are consistent with best practices will operate from a client-centred perspective, valuing and responding to the client's own desires and preferences related to employment. Yet, addressing motivational issues that can cloud client choice and weaken commitment and follow through with vocational plans requires understanding and skill on the part of the service provider.

This chapter focuses on motivational issues that can impact the employment outcomes of people with mental illness and challenge vocational service delivery. The chapter focuses on motivation for employment in the community labour force, but in no way is intended to negate the value of other productivity roles such as being a student or a community volunteer. Rather, the focus on employment emerges from a concern that a significant number of people with mental illness have a latent desire for employment that, to date, has been poorly addressed within our mental health services and systems.

In this chapter, motivation is defined as those processes, related to employment, which can (1) arouse and instigate vocational behaviour, (2) give direction and purpose to vocational behaviour, (3) allow vocational behaviours to persist and (4) lead to choosing or preferring a particular vocational behaviour (adapted from Wlodkowski, 1999). This is a broad, comprehensive definition of motivation related to employment, but each of its components is important. The definition suggests that motivation for employment can be expressed in many ways, including, for example, a lack of desire for employment, a lack of focus to vocational behaviours, inconsistent or sporadic vocational behaviours and difficulties with commitment to the responsibilities of employment.

This chapter will examine:

• Motivational issues that can hinder vocational recovery
• Approaches that vocational service providers can use to promote motivation for employment

Background

Involvement in productive activities that contribute to the socio-economic well-being and prosperity of the individual and the community is considered fundamental to full citizenship and social participation. Employment from the perspective of citizenship is viewed as both a personal right (that comes with considerable benefits) and as a responsibility. People who experience mental illness are no less tied to these ideals of employment than other members of the general public. Yet their high rates of unemployment and the difficulties they can experience in work are indicative of many recurring factors that challenge their full community participation.

There is consistent evidence to support that people with mental illness place a high value on employment, and given the opportunity would like to work (Crowther et al., 2001; Dunn et al., 2008). Yet, despite their interest in employment, a significant number of people with mental illness are not actively engaged in the community labour force by seeking employment (Waghorn & Lloyd, 2005) or by expressing the motivation for employment that is required for involvement with many vocational support services (Macias et al., 2001).

For practitioners, this inconsistency between population-level information about the desire for employment and the actual intentions of individual clients suggests the presence of a moral dilemma facing service providers. On the one hand, client-centred practice is a hallmark of contemporary rehabilitation practice (Law et al., 1995). In client-centred practice, clients are recognised as the experts of their own lives, and the identification of and planning for goals starts with their own interests and desires. From this perspective, the practitioner can take an individual client's apparent lack of interest in employment at face value and eliminate employment as a potential goal. Yet, the evidence indicates that people with mental illness, like the general public, value employment. This suggests the need to consider more closely, the many experiences and influences that might have shaped attitudes, decisions and perseverance related to working. In the end, the conscientious practitioner must carefully consider if a lack of expressed desire to work might originate from the inability to see a future where employment is a viable option.

Building the hope and motivation of people with serious mental illness for important social activities and roles is an important component of recovery-oriented services that are meant to enable life beyond the constraints posed by the illness (Anthony, 1993). Yet services focused on improving the employment outcomes of people with serious mental illness have tended not to directly focus on the motivational issues that might serve as barriers to people in accessing and persevering with employment efforts. For example, the evidence-based Individual Placement and Support Model has historically been offered to those individuals who have a desire for competitive employment (Bond, 2004). Concerns have been raised about the number of individuals who might be denied access to these vocational services because they lack the self-confidence and work experiences consistent with a decision to work (Macias et al., 2001). Recognising this issue, Drake and Bond (2008) in a recent publication focusing on the future of supported employment services identified the need for innovation in strategies to enhance the motivation of people with mental illness in order to improve upon the considerable success that evidence-based models of supported employment have been able to achieve.

Motivation is a complex phenomenon. Issues of motivation for employment emerging in the context of mental illness reflect a range of interacting factors. This can make it difficult to isolate and define particularly problematic issues and to develop approaches and interventions that are likely to be effective. The following section describes several distinct factors that have been associated with the motivational problems, organised using the conceptual framework of the Person-Environment-Occupation model (PEO; Strong et al., 1999). The PEO is an ecological model that serves as a practical analytic tool to assist practitioners in evaluating, planning and intervening for complex occupational issues. Applied to issues related to motivation for employment, the framework facilitates systematic identification of personal factors – those factorsintrinsic to the individual thatenable or restrict motivation for employment; environmental factors – physical, social, cultural or institutional factors external to the individual that influence motivation for employment; and occupations – defined as tasks and activities that have value and meaning to individuals and society.

Personal factors

Does the person experience the affective pleasures and emotional rewards of participating in employment and work-related activities?

Affective experiences are central to focused and sustained participation in activities and roles such as work. For example, a person may experience a range of emotions over the course of a day of working (interest, pleasure, dissatisfaction, anger, feelings of accomplishment), but sustaining employment is enhanced when affective experiences are balanced towards those that are felt as positive and rewarding. Many people with mental illness experience disturbances in affect that can compromise their motivation for daily life activities and social relationships. This was an important issue for Dion, the fellow presented in the opening paragraph of this chapter.

The negative symptoms of schizophrenia include apathy, affective flattening, avolition and a disturbed sense of joy/pleasure, and these can translate into problems with motivation for work (Bond & Meyer, 1999; Cook & Razzano, 2000; Lysaker & Bell, 1995). Research has demonstrated a relationship between the presence of these negative symptoms and poorer employment outcomes (Razzano et al., 2005; Tsang et al., 2000). Velligan et al. (2006) point out that the neurophysiological processes underlying these negative symptoms do not necessarily rob the individual of valuing important social roles and activities, such as working, but rather they appear to compromise the effort directed towards them.

People with depression can experience a troubling lack of interest in daily activities, including employment, which influences their drive and initiative for participation. A negative self and world view is another common feature of depression, which affects the optimism and self-esteem needed to engage in employment. Symptoms associated with anxiety can include apprehensiveness and lack of initiative that can be expressed as limited motivation for work.

There have been significant advancements in the pharmacological treatment of mental illness, yet the impact of some of these treatments on motivation continues to be a concern. For example, medications designed to treat psychosis have been effective in treating positive symptoms, such as hallucinations, but less effective in reducing the negative symptoms associated with amotivation. Although it has been hoped that the newer generation of atypical anti-psychotic medications would better manage these negative symptoms, research has not consistently supported this finding (Gardner et al., 2005). These atypical anti-psychotic medications do appear to reduce the risk of adverse neurological side effects that could interfere with an individual following through with a desire for employment. They have, however, been associated with other side effects, in particular significant weight gain (Gardner et al., 2005), that might undermine motivation for social roles such as employment.

Does the person evaluate his or her skills and competencies to be consistent with success in employment?

Employment makes significant performance demands on workers. It comes with expectations that individuals will be able to fulfil task demands associated with the production of specific goods or services, social demands related to social interactions at work and also the performance of a range of work behaviours that facilitate the function of the work organization. In addition, the individual with a mental illness who decides to pursue employment is challenged by many other demands. The person might, for example, be engaged in illness self-management while working, be faced with negotiating how to best disclose mental illness in the work context and perhaps be faced with learning compensatory strategies to manage the impact of cognitive problems on the job (Krupa, 2004; Krupa et al., 2008). From this perspective of 'extra effort', the person with mental illness engaged in employment might be viewed as demonstrating a very high level of motivation.

Motivation for employment can be negatively affected when the individual perceives (accurately or inaccurately) that his or her own abilities, aptitudes and strengths are not up to meeting work-related demands. This perception renders him or her vulnerable to anticipation of failure and rejection and ultimately compromises the extent to which the individual will act on the desire to work. Poor self-efficacy has long been associated with a negative influence on the effort and perseverance that people will apply when faced with challenges in daily activities (Bandura, 1977), but has only recently been applied to understand career decision-making and behaviours in people with mental illness (Corbiere et al., 2004; Renegold et al., 1999; Waghorn et al., 2007)

Self-efficacy for employment when living with mental illness can be compromised in several ways. Given that mental illness can disrupt education and early work experiences, the individual may perceive personal disadvantage relative to other workers in competition for valued jobs. The individual may perceive that his or her current experience of mental health will impact performance at work or that specific capacities have been affected by mental illness and judge the potential for meeting work demands negatively. An individual who has experienced an exacerbation of acute mental illness following a return to work may be guarded about his or her ability to manage both the illness and employment.

Environmental factors

Does the individual evaluate his or her material resources as consistent with success in employment?

Since one of the main motivations for employment is to receive the income required to purchase important material goods, it is easy to forget that working itself requires a considerable outlay of resources. Personal expenses related to working can include the costs of transportation, clothing and gear that is appropriate to the specific job position, and the finances to participate in social interactions on the job in a way that promotes acceptance and inclusion. The bottom line is that in employment, people need to spend money to make money.

The high levels of poverty among people with mental illness are well known, and have been associated with their high levels of unemployment and low levels of income provided by government financial assistance schemes (Cook, 2006; Nordt et al., 2007). Lack of financial means is likely to enter into the employment decisions of people with mental illness (Cook, 2006). Unfortunately, there has been little systematic study of the impact of poverty on working and the evidence has largely been anecdotal. Stories collected from the field include the case of a gentleman who decided that he could not persist in employment because he could not afford the increased grocery bill that came with work-related physical exertion, the young woman without a vehicle who decided that the job she held was not worth the effort of the hours and half trips on public transport, and a group of consumers who stated that they could not hope to secure employment without the means to pay for proper dental work.

An area that has received attention in the field is the extent to which people with mental illness who are financially supported by government disability benefits are caught in a 'poverty trap' (Cook, 2006) referring to the way these income structures act as disincentives to employment. These disincentives include the development of an internalised label of 'retired' from the community-based workforce, fear of losing financial security, complicated administrative processes that leave the individual feeling financially vulnerable, and concerns about the loss of medical coverage provided by income support schemes (Turton, 2001; Leff & Warner, 2006).

Does the individual evaluate his or her social resources as supportive of employment?

The extent to which people in the social network are supportive of employment has been associated with the individual's intention to secure and sustain employment. It is believed that social support is important both in affirming that employment is an important and worthwhile endeavour and in enabling the perception that people are available to facilitate coping with work-related challenges (Kanfer et al., 2001; Vinokur & Caplan, 2006).

The social networks of people with mental illness can be relatively small and have weak support systems (Biegal et al., 1995). This means that the individual with mental illness might have fewer social supports to draw on to enable their motivation to work. The extent to which the individual's employment history is reflective of marginalisation from the community workforce, vocational service providers can expect to see limited opportunities to capitalise on existing employment networks as a means to support the individual's efforts to secure and keep work. For those in employment, the quality of the relationships with co-workers and supervisors might influence the individual's commitment to deal with work-related challenges.

An area of particular concern is the extent to which social supports actually communicate the view that employment is a worthwhile and feasible goal to the person living with mental illness. Families and friends may actively discourage employment for a variety of reasons, such as concerns about disturbing income support payments and uncertainty about the extent to which employment might represent an overwhelming stressor (Krupa et al., 2008; Leff & Warner, 2006). People with mental illness will also receive mixed messages about employment from mental health service providers who operate in a system where employment is not considered a priority in service delivery and who may not have up-to-date information about the potential for employment with proven supports (Krupa, 2004; Leff & Warner, 2006).

How does the social stigma of mental illness influence the individual's self-view?

Stigma is considered one of the most profound barriers to the employment of people with mental illness. The extent to which stigma, or negative labelling, is accepted and internalised by people with mental illness will influence employment outcomes by decreasing self-esteem, self-efficacy, hope and ultimately the motivation for actively seeking out and securing work (Lysaker et al., 2007). Indeed, current conceptualisations of internalised stigma have highlighted both secrecy and withdrawal as coping strategies used to deal with the expectation of stigma and discrimination (Vauth et al., 2007)

Employment is a particularly complex context for an individual to manage information presented to the public about the illness. With its formal job descriptions, ongoing demands for productivity and explicit behavioural organization, employment may challenge the individual's ability to be able to conceal the mental illness and be a considerable source of stress with regard to what and how to disclose illness-related information.

Occupational factors

Are there opportunities for the person to participate in work that is both personally and socially valued and meaningful?

One of the defining features of contemporary vocational service delivery has been the focus on employment as a community resource – a resource that should be fully accessible to people with mental illness as community citizens (Nelson et al., 2001). In response to this focus, the field has developed models of employment support that have demonstrated considerable success in improving the employment outcomes of people with mental illness. These successes can provide people with mental illness with important evidence that they need to evaluate real work in the community as a viable option. Ongoing concerns remain, however, about the extent to which these work outcomes represent entry-level, low-paying positions with limited opportunities for promotion and career advancement (Baron & Salzer, 2002). Indeed, critiques of these work-related initiatives have highlighted the extent to which employment has been limited to '. . . the Four F's: food, flowers, folding and filth (referring to the stereotypical entry-level positions often offered [to] clients with long-term mental illness: food service, gardening, laundry or clerical work, and janitorial services)' (Corbett, 2003)

Dooley et al. (2000) stress the importance of developing conceptualisations of employment status beyond the simple 'employment/no employment' categories. They suggest that underemployment, referring to a range of adverse employment conditions is important to consider. It can leave people with mental illness at risk for a drift down in occupational status and can be associated with poorer mental health, including lowered self-esteem and an increase in symptoms of depression.

With regard to motivation for employment the salient point is that for the individual with mental illness, employment opportunities will be evaluated with regard to the extent to which they are personally and socially meaningful, rewarding and viable. Ultimately, the extent to which employment opportunities are judged as being below personal expectations will lead to compromising of the motivation for employment.

Approaches to facilitate motivation for employment

Motivation for employment in the context of mental illness has been presented in this chapter as a complex issue influenced by a range of profound and interacting factors. Approaches that will enable the motivation required to secure and sustain employment will be characterised by patience, hopefulness, creativity, comprehensiveness and the integration of evidence-based employment principles and practices that reveal and capitalise on strengths and capacities. While change can be a slow process, it should be remembered that motivation for employment can emerge in unexpected ways and places, and once it emerges it can lead to remarkably rapid and positive changes.

Perhaps one of the best strategies we have to enable in the motivation for work is to continue with the advancement of a range of employment support models and strategies that demonstrate effectiveness in achieving meaningful community employment, and to ensure the accessibility of these to those individuals with mental illness who require them. The positive employment outcomes demonstrated by approaches (such as Individual Placement and Support, community economic initiatives like social businesses and initiatives to affirmatively employ people with mental illness within the mental health system) provide several employment options and send powerful, positive messages about employment potential. They are also designed to assure individuals that their personal support needs will be addressed and thus encourage ongoing motivation for work.

Interestingly, there is some evidence to support the assertive provision of employment support services even when an individual's interest for employment is low. Macias et al. (2001) studied the outcomes of offering employment support services to individuals with serious mental illness who received services from two community-based mental health services. They found that approximately half of those who initially expressed no interest in working used the vocational services and obtained employment. The researchers argue for the routine provision of vocational services integrated within mental health programmes as a means to nurture the motivation for work. It may be that engagement in these work activities provided individuals with the conditions required to stimulate their interest and to counteract negative self-evaluations holding them back from employment.

Unfortunately, there are few practice guidelines and minimal research evidence to offer the vocational service provider who is attending to increasing the motivation for employment of an individual who is living with mental illness. A comprehensive understanding of the factors that are likely contributing to poor motivation is important, providing a foundation for determining which should be specifically targeted by interventions. This is best accomplished within a collaborative and client-centred relationship that contributes to motivational processes by actively engaging the individual as experts in their own needs and preferences. The establishment of the client-centred relationship can be particularly challenging when clients have significant problems with motivation. Vocational service providers need to be aware of their own vulnerability to responding to a client's lack of interest and inconsistent effort towards employment goals with expressions of frustration that can derail the collaborative working alliance.

Motivational interviewing developed initially as a process to facilitate the decrease in substance using behaviours has been adapted within the field of psychiatric rehabilitation to enable a comprehensive process of goal setting (Corrigan et al., 2001). Motivational interviewing systematically engages the individual with mental illness to consider the various advantages and disadvantages of selecting employment as a goal. It offers the service provider opportunities to 'tip the balance' in favour of behaviour change in an empathic and ultimately client-directed therapeutic context.

While the assessment of motivational factors will largely occur as a guided reflection within the therapeutic relationship, a range of relevant and standardised assessments have been developed and may provide focused information to enhance understanding and support vocational counselling and career planning. For example, the Work-related Self-efficacy Scale (Waghorn et al., 2005) is a 37-item scale measuring self-efficacy for people with mental illness in four relevant activity domains consisting of vocational service access and career planning, job acquisition, work-related social skills and general work skills. The Work-related Subjective Experiences Scale is a 38-item measure of personal experiences, often self-reported as barriers to employment (Waghorn et al., 2007). This measure provides information about how a person's affective state is likely to respond to challenging situations such as in a new job. The Barriers to Employment and Coping Self-efficacy Scale (Corbiere et al., 2004) identifies

35 potential barriers to employment and engages individuals in rating their perceived ability to cope with and overcome identified barriers.

Vocational counselling focused on revealing and acting on the individual's personal preferences for employment is consistent with theories of enabling motivation and one of the central principles of providing employment support (Bond, 2004). Concerns about the extent to which people with mental illness may select inappropriate job preferences have not been supported by research evidence, particularly when these preferences are matched with ongoing and individualised employment support (Mueser et al., 2001). Vocational counselling can provide the processes for good decision-making about job preferences, including consideration of a range of important factors such as interests, strengths, aptitudes, work experiences and potential resources.

There has been remarkably little direct attention paid to addressing the affective and emotional disturbances that impact motivation for activities, social experiences and roles such as work. Certainly the vocational service provider will need to work collaboratively with the individual and other health service providers to ensure that decisions about medications and other medical treatments give full consideration to emotion and affect that interferes with motivation. For many people, these troubling affective experiences will be an ongoing concern. Several strategies to address these issues that have been presented in the literature are as follows (Krupa, 1986; Velligan et al., 2006; Wu et al., 2000):

- Provide the client with education about these affective and emotional disturbances to promote their active engagement in management strategies. This education can be extended to family and friends to engage their active involvement in encouraging motivation.
- Identify multiple personal values and reasons that might be developed as a source of motivation for employment. For example, an individual's motivation might emerge from a desire to be seen as a contributing member of society, to contribute financially to family/children, to spend time away from the home or neighbourhood, to meet cultural expectations or to provide structure to an otherwise occupationally vacant day.
- Identify pleasure and emotional well-being as they occur in work-related activities as a means to cue attention to rewarding experiences that might facilitate ongoing motivation.
- Carefully match employment choices to the affective and emotional capacities of the individual.

While the best strategy to overcome issues of self-efficacy influencing employment intervention remains actively engaging individuals in work-related activities with needed supports to build skills and confidence, cognitive-behavioural therapy may be a useful adjunct approach. In an effort to address the negative self-beliefs that compromised work participation and performance, Lysaker et al. (2005) developed and evaluated a group format cognitive-behavioural intervention, the Indianapolis Vocational Intervention Program, to target and alter dysfunctional beliefs about the self. Study results were promising, demonstrating improvements in measures of hopefulness and self-esteem, and better work performance and more weeks at work compared to the group who received employment support alone.

Peer support has also been identified as a strategy to overcome the negative self-views and hopelessness fundamental to low motivation for employment (Cook & Razzano, 2000; Davidson et al., 2006). Interactions with peers with mental illness who have been successful in meaningful and respected employment can enlarge an individual's expectations related to work by foiling negative self-perceptions about personal capacities and potentials. Another benefit of formalised peer-provider and peer-run initiatives is their potential to counteract the public stigma that can interfere with the motivation for employment among all persons with mental illness.

Low motivation for employment emerging from fears of stigmatisation and discrimination will require direct attention to issues of disclosure in the work context. Disclosure counselling and training can focus on informed decision-making about disclosure and strategic planning with regard to the nature of disclosure. For example, disclosure counselling might focus on what specific information to share, with whom the information will be shared, timing of disclosure, developing requests for required accommodations and the benefits and threats of disclosure (Corrigan & Matthews, 2003; Goldberg et al., 2005). An integral component of dealing with disclosure will be addressing the individual's acceptance of and personal identity of having a mental illness, whether the individual decided to 'come out' or not. Corrigan and Matthews (2003) identify several positive identities that might be internalised by individuals with serious mental illness.

Advocacy and lobbying strategies are required to address policies that create economic disincentives to employment for individuals with mental illness. Yet, there are strategies that vocational service providers can use to help decrease any individual's experience of financial insecurity and constraints. Benefits counselling focuses on developing an individual's understanding of complex government financial benefits and using this information for informed decision-making related to employment. A recent study demonstrated that those receiving specialised benefits counselling increased their earnings (Tremblay et al., 2006).

Conclusions

Issues related to motivation have the potential to interfere with vocational recovery. Addressing motivational problems is challenging because there can be many complex and long-standing factors contributing to the problem. The service provider can be caught in trying to simultaneously respect a client's choices while remaining determined to enlarge the individual's self-view and expectations through meaningful social roles such as employment. The worth of these efforts is supported by personal narratives of people who, in the process of recovery from mental illness, have moved from passive participants in life to active engagement in fulfilling occupations such as employment. Readers of this chapter are encouraged to visit the writings of Patricia Deegan (1996) whose personal testimonies so profoundly illustrate this process. The strategies to address motivational problems that are described in this chapter provide a range of possibilities that can be implemented within a collaborative client–provider relationship and integrated within a vocational system providing access to evidence-based vocational services.

References

Anthony, W. (1993). Recovery: the guiding vision of the mental health service system in the 1990's. *Psychiatric Rehabilitation Journal, 16*, 11–23.

Bandura, A. (1977). Self-efficacy: toward a unifying theory of behavioral change. *Psychological Review, 84*, 191–215.

Baron, R., & Salzer, M. (2002). Accounting for unemployment among people with mental illness. *Behavioral Sciences and the Law, 20*, 585–599.

Biegal, D.E., Tracy, E.M., & Song, L. (1995). Barriers to social network interventions with persons with serious mental illness: a survey of mental health case managers. *Community Mental Health Journal, 31*, 335–349.

Bond, G. (2004). Supported employment: evidence for an evidence-based practice. *Psychiatric Rehabilitation Journal, 27*, 347–359.

Bond, G.R., & Meyer, P.S. (1999). The role of medications in the employment of people with schizophrenia. *Journal of Rehabilitation, 65*, 9–16.

Cook, J. (2006). Employment barriers for persons with psychiatric disabilities: update of a report for the President's Commission. *Psychiatric Services, 57*, 1391–1405.

Cook, J.A., & Razzano, L.A. (2000). Vocational rehabilitation for people with psychiatric disability. *American Rehabilitation, 20*, 2–12.

Corbett, G. (2003). Psychiatric impairment and vocational considerations. *Rehabilitation Review, 19*, 4–7.

Corbiere, M., Mercier, C., & Lesage, A. (2004). Perceptions of barriers to employment, coping efficacy and career search efficacy in people with mental illness. *Journal of Career Assessment, 12*, 460–478.

Corrigan, P.W., & Matthews, A.K. (2003). Stigma and disclosure: implications for coming out of the closet. *Journal of Mental Health, 12*, 235–248.

Corrigan, P.W., McCracken, S.G., & Holmes, E.P. (2001). Motivational interviews as goal assessment for persons with psychiatric disability. *Community Mental Health Journal, 37*, 113–122.

Crowther, R.E., Marshall, M., Bond, G.R., & Huxley, P. (2001). Helping people with severe mental illness to obtain work: systematic reviews. *British Medical Journal, 322*(7280), 204–208.

Davidson, L., Chinman, M., Sells, D., & Row, M. (2006). Peer support among adults with serious mental illness: a report from the field. *Schizophrenia Bulletin, 32,* 443–450.

Deegan, P. (1996). Recovery and the conspiracy of hope. Presented at the Sixth Annual Mental Health Conference of Australia and New Zealand, Brisbane, Australia. Available at: http://www.namiscc.org/newsletters/February02/PatDeegan.htm (accessed 15 November 2008).

Dooley, D., Prause, J., & Ham-Rowbottom, K.A. (2000). Underemployment and depression: longitudinal relationships. *Journal of Health and Social Behavior, 41,* 421–436.

Drake, R.E., & Bond, G.R. (2008). The future of supported employment for people with severe mental illness. *Psychiatric Rehabilitation Journal, 31,* 367–376.

Dunn, E.C., Wewiorski, N.J., & Rogers, E.S. (2008). The meaning and importance of employment to people in recovery from serious mental illness: results of a qualitative study. *Psychiatric Rehabilitation Journal, 32,* 59–62.

Gardner, D.M., Baldessarini, R.J., & Waraich, P. (2005). Modern antipsychotic drugs: a critical overview. *Canadian Medical Association Journal, 172,* 1703–1711.

Goldberg, S.G., Killeen, M.B., & O'Day, B. (2005). The disclosure conundrum: how people with psychiatric disabilities navigate employment. *Psychology, Public Policy and Law, 11,* 463–500.

Kanfer, R., Wanberg, C.R., & Kantrowitz, T.M. (2001). Job search and employment: a personality-motivational analysis and meta-analytic review. *Journal of Applied Psychology, 86,* 837–855.

Krupa, T. (1986). The pleasure deficit in schizophrenia. *Occupational Therapy in Mental Health, 6,* 65–78.

Krupa, T. (2004). Employment, recovery and schizophrenia: integrating health and disorder at work. *Psychiatric Rehabilitation Journal, 28,* 8–15.

Krupa, T., Woodside, H., & Pocock, K. (2008). Activity and social participation in first episode psychosis. *Early Intervention in Psychiatry,* 2(Suppl.), 66.

Law, M., Baptiste, S., & Mills, J. (1995). Client-centred practice: what does it mean and does it make a difference? *Canadian Journal of Occupational Therapy, 62,* 250–257.

Leff, J., & Warner, R. (2006). *Social Inclusion and Serious Mental Illness.* Cambridge, UK: Cambridge University Press.

Lysaker, P., & Bell, M. (1995). Negative symptoms and vocational impairment in schizophrenia: repeated measurements of work performance over six months. *Acta Psychiatrica Scandinavica, 91,* 205–208.

Lysaker, P.H., Bond, G., Davis, L.W., Bryson, G.J., & Bell, M.D. (2005). Enhanced cognitive-behavioral therapy for vocational rehabilitation in schizophrenia: effects on hope and work. *Journal of Rehabilitation Research and Development, 42,* 673–682.

Lysaker, P.H., Roe, D., & Yanos, P.T. (2007). Toward understanding the insight paradox: internalized stigma moderates the association between insight and social functioning, hope and self-esteem among people with schizophrenia spectrum disorders. *Schizophrenia Bulletin, 33,* 192–199.

Macias, C., DeCarlo, L.T., Wang, Q., Frey, J., & Barreira, P. (2001). Work interest as a predictor of competitive employment: policy implications for psychiatric rehabilitation. *Administration and Policy in Mental Health, 28,* 279–297.

Mueser, K.T., Becker, D.R., & Wolfe, R. (2001). Supported employment, job preferences, job tenure and satisfaction. *Journal of Mental Health, 10,* 411–417.

Nelson, G., Lord, J., & Ochocka, J. (2001). *Shifting the Paradigm in Community Mental Health: Towards Empowerment and Community.* Toronto: University of Toronto Press.

Nordt, C., Müller, B., Rössler, W., & Lauber, C. (2007). Predictors and course of vocational status, income, and quality of life in people with severe mental illness: a naturalistic study. *Social Sciences and Medicine*, 65, 1420–1429.

Razzano, L.A., Cook, J., Burke-Miller, J.K., Mueser, K.T., Pickett-Schenk, S.A., Grey, D.D., Goldberg, R.W., Blyler, C.R., Gold, P.B., Leff, H.S., Lehman, A., Shafer, M., Blankertz, L.E., McFarlane, W.R., Toprac, M.G., & Carey, M.A. (2005). Clinical factors associated with employment among people with severe mental illness. *The Journal of Nervous and Mental Disease*, 193, 705–713.

Renegold, M., Sherman, M.F., & Fenzel, M. (1999). Getting back to work: self-efficacy as a predictor of employment outcome. *Psychiatric Rehabilitation Journal*, 22, 361–367.

Strong, S., Rigby, P., Stewart, D., Law, M., Letts, L., & Cooper, B. (1999). Application of the person–environment–occupation model: a practical tool. *Canadian Journal of Occupational Therapy*, 66, 122–133.

Tremblay, T., Smith, J., Xie, H., & Drake, R. (2006). Effect of benefits counseling services on employment outcomes for people with psychiatric disabilities. *Psychiatric Services*, 57, 816–821.

Tsang, H., Lam, P., Ng, B., & Leung, O. (2000). Predictors of employment outcome for people with psychiatric disabilities: a review of the literature since the mid '80's. *Journal of Rehabilitation*, 66, 19–25.

Turton, N. (2001). Welfare benefits and work disincentives. *Journal of Mental Health*, 20, 285–300.

Vauth, R., Kleim, B., Wirtz, M., & Corrigan, PW. (2007). Self-efficacy and empowerment as outcomes of self-stigmatizing and coping in schizophrenia. *Psychiatric Research*, 150, 71–80.

Velligan, D.I., Kern, R.S., & Gold, J.M. (2006). Cognitive rehabilitation for schizophrenia and the putative role of motivation and expectancies. *Schizophrenia Bulletin*, 32, 474–485.

Vinokur, A., & Caplan, R.D. (2006). Attitudes and social support: determinants of job-seeking behavior and well-being among the unemployed. *Journal of Applied Social Psychology*, 17, 1007–1024.

Waghorn, G., Chant, D., & King, R. (2005). Work-related self-efficacy among community residents with psychiatric disabilities. *Psychiatric Rehabilitation Journal*, 29, 105–113.

Waghorn, G.R., Chant, D.C., & King, R. (2007). Work-related subjective experiences, work-related self-efficacy, and career learning among people with psychiatric disabilities. *American Journal of Psychiatric Rehabilitation*, 10, 275–300.

Waghorn, G., & Lloyd, C. (2005). The employment of people with mental illness. *Australian e-Journal for the Advancement of Mental Health*, 4(2, Suppl.).

Wlodkowski, R.J. (1999). *Enhancing Adult Motivation to Learn: A Comprehensive Guide for Teaching all Adults*. San Francisco: Jossey-Bass Publishers.

Wu, C., Chen, S., & Grossman, J. (2000). Facilitating intrinsic motivation in clients with mental illness. *Occupational Therapy in Mental Health*, 16, 1–14.

Chapter 7

THERAPEUTIC ALLIANCE IN VOCATIONAL REHABILITATION

Frank P. Deane, Trevor P. Crowe and Lindsay G. Oades

Chapter overview

The chapter begins by providing a brief description of the components thought to be important in the therapeutic relationship and in developing a strong therapeutic or working alliance. Many decades of research have established that a good therapeutic alliance is related to better treatment outcomes for people engaged in psychotherapy. However, there has been relatively little of this research which has focused on individuals with severe mental illnesses such as schizophrenia. A brief review of these studies indicates 'promising' findings with regard to the link between therapeutic alliance and more positive treatment outcomes, but it is argued that a strength-based emphasis in treatment may be particularly important for those with severe mental illnesses. A detailed review is then provided of the research related specifically to the role of therapeutic alliance in vocational rehabilitation contexts. Given the relatively small number of studies focusing on vocational outcomes, this starts with a review of four studies comprising individuals with traumatic brain injury and is followed by a description of the two studies that used participants with mental illness. Again, the data are promising and together suggest a positive relationship between stronger therapeutic alliance and a range of more positive vocational outcomes. This is followed by a description of the main measures used to assess therapeutic alliance and an overview of the key components thought to strengthen the alliance. Finally, the chapter finishes with a section describing how to therapeutically manage difficulties in the alliance. These are described as 'strains and ruptures', and the chapter concludes with strategies for identifying and resolving these fluctuations in the quality and strength of the therapeutic alliance.

Components of therapeutic relationship

Rogers (1957) suggested that therapists require the personal qualities of accurate empathy, non-possessive warmth and unconditional acceptance, and genuineness to establish a quality therapeutic relationship. It was thought that this therapeutic relationship would in turn facilitate a positive change. This

conceptualisation of these relationship factors was broadly thought to constitute what is known as 'bond' in therapy and each of these elements are briefly
described below.

Accurate empathy

There is some debate regarding the meaning of accurate empathy, but it is
essentially a cognitive and affective state that involves recognising and engaging
with the client's affect or cognition and reflecting this back to them from
moment to moment (Duan & Hill, 1996). Thus, a counsellor needs to be able
to imagine or understand the client's experience and then to accurately reflect
this back. This reflection could be a verbal statement or affective (emotional)
response. Accurate empathy involves listening carefully to what clients say,
how they say it and being aware of the nonverbal information that might also
help understand their experience. Trying to imagine or understand someone
else's experience can be difficult. While practitioners can draw on their own
reactions in similar circumstances in order to get a sense of a client's view, they
cannot presume that their experiences and reactions are the same as those of
their clients. In this respect, they need to remain open to different perspectives.

Non-possessive warmth and unconditional acceptance

Non-possessive warmth refers to caring, respect, support and valuing the client
without attempting to control them (Todd & Bohart, 1994). Part of this stance
is accepting and respecting the client's autonomy. Unconditional acceptance
refers to the ability to listen and respond to others without being judgemental
or disapproving.

Genuineness

Genuineness refers to the ability of a clinician to be honest, open and authentic
in his or her interactions with clients. Genuineness is reflected in the consistency
between how a person acts and how they think and feel (Todd & Bohart, 1994).

Empathy, warmth, acceptance and genuineness are generally considered important clinician characteristics for the development of a good therapeutic
relationship. However, the client–therapist working relationship involves reciprocity and this is captured in the broader term *therapeutic alliance*.

Therapeutic alliance

Therapeutic or working alliance is a more specific term that was described by
Bordin (1979) as comprising a mutual understanding and an agreement about
goals, an agreement on the necessary tasks to move toward these goals and the

establishment of a bond between the partners involved in the work (typically the health care provider and the client). Tasks are distinguished from goals in that they involve specific activities that are undertaken either during the session or out of session to facilitate change. They can also be proposals for client action such as between session homework activities such as 'making a telephone call to prospective employers' or 'writing out a list of strengths that might be attractive to prospective employers'. Negotiation between counsellor and client around goals and tasks is considered integral to building alliance (Bordin, 1994). Bond in the therapeutic relationship is consistent with the core characteristics described by Rogers (1957), and Bordin (1994) described this as 'expressed and felt in terms of liking, trusting, respect for each other' and 'a sense of common commitment and shared understanding in the activity' (p. 16). The bond in the therapeutic relationship is often considered the 'glue' that helps maintain the partnership through what can be difficult and challenging personal demands on clients and therapists in therapy over time. To summarise, the following characteristics have been suggested as common components of therapeutic alliance: the client's positive affective relationship with the therapist, the client's capacity to purposefully work in therapy, the therapist's empathic understanding and involvement and the client–therapist agreement on the goals and tasks of therapy (Gaston, 1990).

Therapeutic alliance and treatment outcomes

There is a substantial body of evidence to support the role of therapeutic alliance factors in treatment outcome. However, relatively little of this research has been with clients with severe mental illness and as we will see in the next section, even less of this has been completed in the context of vocational rehabilitation.

A meta-analytic review of 79 studies over an 18-year span found a minority of studies (23%) included more severely disordered clients (i.e. psychotic or severe personality disorders) (Martin et al., 2000). The meta-analysis found a moderate positive relationship between therapeutic alliance and outcome (overall weighted correlation of .22). No other moderator variables influenced the alliance–outcome relationship, which is consistent with the hypothesis that the alliance is therapeutic, in and of itself, and regardless of other psychological interventions (Martin et al., 2000).

Research on the role and impact of therapeutic alliance in working with individuals with chronic and recurring psychotic mental illnesses such as schizophrenia is relatively limited but there has been increasing interest amongst such groups (Couture et al., 2006; McCabe & Priebe, 2004; Priebe & McCabe, 2006).

At a general level, the therapeutic alliance has been found to be related to treatment adherence (including medications) and other outcomes amongst patients with schizophrenia (e.g. Gehrs & Goering, 1994; Svensson & Hansson, 1999). For example, in a study of clients with non-chronic schizophrenia, it was found that the alliance-predicted medication adherence was negatively related to psychopathology, frequency of positive symptoms and treatment dropout. The alliance also predicted improved social functioning and illness acceptance, and accounted for more outcome variance than social class, intelligence, insight, baseline symptom level, optimism, motivation to change and level of pre-morbid functioning (Frank & Gunderson, 1990).

A descriptive review that focused on studies of alliance outcome in community psychiatry and case management located five studies assessing the relationship in these contexts (Howgego et al., 2003). Most of the clients in these studies had severe mental health problems such as schizophrenia, and the review concluded that there was 'minimal' but 'encouraging' evidence that stronger case manager–client therapeutic relationships resulted in improved outcomes. The authors suggested that this population may require a longer time period to develop a positive alliance and that the social or relationship competence of clients may influence the formation of the alliance. The issue of specific skills to address alliance issues amongst clients with severe mental illnesses such as schizophrenia has also been raised by other authors (e.g. Priebe & McCabe, 2006). Currently, there is little empirical research to support the notion that there are different techniques that might be needed to impact on the therapeutic alliance amongst this group compared to other diagnostic groups. Until such data are available, therapists should endeavour to bring the attributes and skills that promote a strong working alliance in any psychotherapeutic relationship (e.g. Ackerman & Hilsenroth, 2003). However, our experience working with individuals who have severe mental illnesses, which are often of long duration and fluctuating course, does provide us with anecdotal evidence that specific stances in relation to rehabilitation are helpful to the therapeutic relationship. A very common theme amongst people with severe mental illness is the loss of hope that often accompanies many years of struggle with the illness. This is exacerbated by stigma and social exclusion. Consequently, we strongly endorse a strengths-based approach and an emphasis on building hope through exploration of values, clarification of a recovery vision, establishment of goals and specific action plans to achieve these goals.

Importance of strengths-based approaches

In clinical contexts and in general life, it is common for people to focus on problems, weaknesses or deficits. This phenomenon has been referred to as 'bad is stronger than good' (Baumeister et al., 2001). Vocational rehabilitation is no exception in this regard. If problems and deficits are the sole focus, this is likely to impact on the rehabilitation alliance, eroding confidence and self-belief, and thus leading the person to a form of 'contraction' or withdrawal. Focusing on strengths, however, can help the person build confidence and hope, buffer against being overwhelmed in the face of challenges and difficulties, and increase their motivation to engage in their rehabilitation and recovery. Confidence and hope are the key pillars of recovery, and if they can be increased by exploring strengths within the working relationship, the relationship itself can be strengthened. This is important as the alliance between the worker and the client can be viewed as the holding framework within which the risk taking of therapeutic work can occur. In this regard the alliance should represent a safe psychological space for the person. Safe places are a fundamental need to support recovery and growth.

Linley and Harrington (2006a) define strength as 'the natural capacity for behaving, thinking or feeling in a way that allows optimal functioning and performance in the pursuit of valued outcomes'. Everybody has strengths and if we are looking for them we will find them. One place to start is to recall memories and feelings associated with achievements or positive actions. It is also important to recognise that strengths are not just talents. They include memories or situations when people have been able to put their core values into action. This allows people to draw on memories when their confidence needs a boost. Strengths can also be social supports, safe and meaningful places and other resources. In effect, strengths are those things that keep the person strong and will often perform a function of confirming the person's preferred identity and desired place within the world.

In terms of building a therapeutic or working relationship with the person, finding common ground to build a conversation is helpful, but exploring the person's strengths, hopes and desires also helps in terms of increasing engagement and ownership of the recovery plan. The rehabilitation relationship in this regard may be conceptualised as a form of 'strengths coaching' (Linley & Harrington, 2006b). The focus remains on human potential and positive consumer attributes. Details of a structured approach to exploring values, establishing a recovery vision, goal and action planning has been elaborated elsewhere as the Collaborative Recovery Model (Clarke et al., 2006; Crowe et al., 2006; Oades et al., 2005). This approach has a strong focus on strengths, which is driven by the belief that the quality of the working relationship is improved by placing it in the context of a focus on client's strengths.

Therapeutic alliance and vocational rehabilitation outcomes

In this section, the few empirical studies of the relationship between therapeutic alliance and vocational rehabilitation outcomes are reviewed in sufficient detail to allow consideration of the strengths, weakness and implications of these studies. Although there have been many studies that have assessed variables that influence successful employment outcomes, only relatively recently has there been research related to the effects of the relationship between counsellors and clients on outcomes. One of the first studies used data from a telephone-administered questionnaire with 2732 vocational rehabilitation clients from 1999 to 2000 (Lustig et al., 2002). The researchers developed a 9-item 'Working Alliance Survey' guided by Bordin's definition of working alliance (bond, goals, tasks) and expert ratings to refine items. They also included measures of the clients' view of their future employment prospects and satisfaction with their current job if they had one. Slightly more than half of the sample was male (56%) and most respondents were employed (67%). Respondents had a range of primary disabilities, with 33% having chronic medical conditions, 27% ($n = 727$) having psychiatric disorders, 19% mobility and orthopaedic impairments, 11% mental retardation and the remaining 10% visual, hearing or traumatic brain impairment. Comparisons between the employed and unemployed groups revealed that a significantly higher proportion of those in the unemployed group had a psychiatric disability. Comparison of the employed and unemployed groups revealed significantly weaker working alliance in the unemployed group compared to the employed group (effect size of $d = .73$). Stronger working alliance was associated with higher levels of satisfaction with the current job ($r = .15, p < .001$). For both employed and unemployed groups, working alliance was also significantly correlated with clients' views of future employment prospects ($r = .51$ and $.52$ respectively). The authors concluded that 'rehabilitation counselors may be able to improve outcomes by facilitating a strong working alliance with their clients' (Lustig et al., 2002, p. 30). However, there were several limitations to the study that suggested caution with this conclusion. First, in the context of the current chapter, only 27% of the sample had a psychiatric disability as their primary disability. Second, contact was attempted with over 10 000 clients, and only 46% were able to be contacted and completed the questionnaires. Of this 46%, only 57% of the completed questionnaires were useable (e.g. due to missing data). It is unclear to what extent these selection issues biased the sample. The measure of therapeutic alliance was developed by the authors but has very limited reliability and validity data. Finally, the data are cross-sectional and predominantly correlational, which prevents any causal conclusions being drawn. For example, it is possible that those who find employment retrospectively view the therapeutic relationship more positively because they are employed. Still, this study establishes that there is some relationship between therapeutic alliance and employment outcomes.

Therapeutic alliance and rehabilitation for traumatic brain injury

Several studies with adults who were receiving rehabilitation for traumatic brain injury also provide relevant data regarding the role of therapeutic alliance on vocational outcomes. A subsequent study to Lustig et al. (2002) used the same

telephone interview method and assessed working alliance and vocational rehabilitation outcomes amongst 49 adult clients who had traumatic brain injury
(Lustig et al., 2003). Slightly more than half (53%) were unemployed and most
of the sample were male (63%). Those in the employed group had significantly stronger working alliance (9-item Working Alliance Survey) compared
to the unemployed group. For the employed clients only, working alliance was
significantly correlated with their view of their future employment prospects
($r = .49$) but not with current job satisfaction. For unemployed clients, stronger
working alliance was associated with a more positive view of future employment prospects ($r = .51$). Overall, this study supported the earlier findings by
Lustig et al. (2002), confirming the relationship between client's perceptions of
working alliance with their vocational counsellor and more optimistic views of
future employment. However, it also suffered the same limitations as the earlier
study.

Other research teams have provided further evidence for the link between
working alliance and subsequent employment (Schonberger et al., 2006b).
Participants were 98 adult patients undergoing post-acute neuropsychological rehabilitation in a brain injury programme in Copenhagen. During the
programme, two expert raters (neuropsychologist and physiotherapist) judged
working alliance using four items adapted for the study. The items assessed the
percentage of client attendance, quality of verbal agreement between therapist
and client as to the course of action, client appreciation of accomplishments
and services, and client engagement. Clients received a dichotomous working
alliance rating based on these four elements and were categorised as having
'poor or fair' or 'good or excellent' alliance. Follow-up of the clients occurred
between 2 months and 3 years after programme completion ($M = 16$ months).
At this time, occupational status was determined and unemployed clients were
compared to those who had some form of competitive or voluntary work.

The percentage of clients rated as having 'good or excellent' alliance was 59
and 46% for each of the two raters. Both raters agreed that 35% of clients
had good or excellent alliance and 30% had poor or fair alliance. For both
raters a significantly higher proportion of clients who were employed had
'good/excellent' alliance compared to those who were unemployed. The raters'
working alliance ratings were significantly related to employment at follow-up.
Limitations of the study included the measure of working alliance which was
not clearly consistent with or explicitly derived from models of alliance (e.g.
Bordin). There was also low interrater agreement and internal consistency on
the alliance measure. Further, the authors noted that alliance ratings were completed retrospectively, so that raters' knowledge of client's outcomes may have
biased their ratings (Schonberger et al., 2006b).

Schonberger et al. (2006a) subsequently addressed most of these limitations
by collecting alliance ratings prospectively in a sample of 86 clients attending a
brain injury rehabilitation programme. The short form of the Working Alliance

Inventory (WAI; Tracey & Kokotovic, 1989) was completed by both clients and therapists at 2, 6, 10 and 14 weeks into the programme and then again at the end of the programme. It was found that task, bond and the total WAI score for therapist ratings significantly improved over time. However, there were no significant changes over time on the client-completed alliance ratings, although clients did rate the therapeutic alliance more positively on all scales and at all time points compared to therapist ratings. Overall, clients and therapists ratings were 'weak-to-moderate' on the total WAI scale (r's ranged from .19 at Time 1 to .45 at Time 4). In general, agreement between client and therapist regarding the strength of the alliance increased over the course of treatment and they tended to converge over time. The authors also hypothesised that a good therapeutic alliance would help increase client's awareness of the impact of their brain injury on their lives (including 'working life'). It was found that the WAI Bond scale was significantly positively correlated with awareness ($r = .28$). The authors concluded:

> The basis of successful work is that the patients experience a good working relationship, including good emotional bond, with their therapist. This is both true for psychotherapeutic work and for cognitive and physical training, because therapeutic success is dependent on patients' engagement and patients' compliance is affected by their experience of a good working alliance and their awareness (p. 453).

A further study of clients with traumatic brain injury attending a rehabilitation programme also assessed alliance, awareness and 'productivity' status (Sherer et al., 2007). The sample comprised 69 clients who were mostly young ($M = 29$ years), male (62%) and had received their injuries following a motor vehicle collision (79%). The California Psychotherapy Alliance Scales (CALPAS; Gaston & Marmar, 1994) was used to assess therapeutic alliance from client, family and clinician perspectives. Similarly, the ratings of awareness were also taken from these three perspectives. Clients were also rated as productive or non-productive at discharge. Those who returned to work or school or were functioning independently as a 'homemaker' were designated as productive, with all others categorised as non-productive. Sixty-two percent were considered productive. Productivity status was predicted by both client and family ratings of therapeutic alliance. However, the direction of this relationship was different for client and family ratings. Stronger family ratings of alliance were associated with a greater likelihood of being in the productive group, whereas higher patient perceptions of therapeutic alliance [were found] to be associated with greater odds of a poor productivity outcome' (p.669). Similarly, stronger therapeutic alliance as rated by clients was associated with greater dropout from the programme. The study failed to find any association between awareness and therapeutic alliance. It was thought that this and the paradoxical finding that higher client ratings of alliance were associated with both higher dropout and poorer productivity may have been due to measures being taken early in treatment (within 2 weeks). It was argued that clients' perceptions of alliance may be more inaccurate early in treatment because there had not been sufficient time to establish a bond and to clarify the goals and tasks that would form part of the treatment and the alliance. However, the study did highlight that family members' early perceptions of therapeutic alliance may be important for longer-term outcomes.

Therapeutic alliance and rehabilitation for severe mental illness

There have been two studies conducted that look at the role of working alliance on vocational outcomes amongst people with severe mental illness. In the first, 305 people with severe mental illness who had received rehabilitation services were contacted by telephone and classified as either employed (36%) or unemployed (64%) (Donnell et al., 2004). They completed the 9-item Working Alliance Survey (as in Lustig et al., 2002, above). Those who were employed provided significantly stronger ratings of therapeutic alliance than those who were unemployed. In both the employed and unemployed groups, working alliance was significantly correlated with their view of future employment prospects ($r = .70$ and $r = .54$ respectively). Employed clients' ratings of alliance were significantly related to their current job satisfaction ($r = .23$), albeit of only modest magnitude. As with their prior study a major limitation of the survey was the measure of therapeutic alliance, which has very limited reliability and validity data.

In a relatively small study involving 26 participants diagnosed with schizophrenia ($n = 12$) or schizoaffective disorder ($n = 14$), the researchers aimed to determine whether therapeutic alliance formed in individual counselling midway through a 26-week vocational rehabilitation programme was related to current and subsequent ratings of work performance (Davis & Lysaker, 2007). Participants were all considered in a stable phase of their illness, with no recent hospitalisations or changes in housing or medications. The observer-rated 12-item version of the WAI was used and multiple blind-raters scored 10 cases in the current study and produced an intraclass correlation of .87, suggesting satisfactory interrater reliability. The Work Behaviour Inventory (WBI; Bryson et al., 1997) was used and involved trained raters directly observing participants' work behaviour and interviews with supervisors. The WBI was completed during Weeks 1, 11 and 23 of work. Satisfactory interrater reliability was found in the study, with intraclass correlations over .82. The type of work was described as involving between 10 and 20 regular hours of work per week in 'entry-level' positions (e.g. housekeeping, medical administration). In the vocational rehabilitation programme, all participants received group or cognitively based individual counselling once a week. The individual counselling sessions focused on dysfunctional beliefs about work and were videotaped to allow for subsequent observer ratings. Using a median split of WAI scores, participants were allocated to a high ($n = 13$) and low ($n = 13$) alliance group. There were no differences between these groups on a range of demographic or symptom-orientated measures. However, there were significant differences between the high and low alliance groups for all five subscales of the WBI. There was a significant improvement for the whole sample on Work Quality and Personal Presentation over time (Weeks 1, 11, 23). However, most notable was a group (high/low alliance) by time interaction, which suggested that those in the high alliance group had higher Work Quality and Cooperativeness scores than the low alliance group at week 23. 'The higher alliance group showed a steady increase over time while the lower alliance group showed initial improvement followed by a decline' (Davis & Lysaker, 2007, p. 355). Although the findings from this study suggest a relationship between alliance and work performance, there are a number of limitations that also need to be considered. The stage of counselling for the assessment of alliance was not clear (i.e. which sessions); the use of median splits to allocate to alliance groups does not have a strong rationale; and the sample was small. Finally, as with other studies assessing alliance and vocational outcomes, the study design does not allow for any conclusions regarding causality.

Summary

There are very few studies that assess the relationship between therapeutic alliance and vocational outcomes in individuals with severe mental illness. However, there are several studies involving people with brain injury which provide additional supporting data. Together these studies suggest a positive relationship between stronger therapeutic alliance and a range of more positive vocational outcomes. Now, there is clearly a need for more longitudinal or experimental designs in more diverse work contexts to allow more causal conclusions to be drawn. There is also a need to clarify the mechanisms and potential mediators of the relationship between alliance and vocational outcomes. For example, does better alliance lead to greater motivation and better compliance with treatment programmes, which in turn lead to better work performance? Or does better work performance occur because a positive alliance models the kinds of work relationships that an individual will experience in the workplace? Until there is clarification of these issues, counsellors should be attentive to the alliance and work to enhance it in counselling contexts. In the future, better understanding the role of alliance in vocational rehabilitation contexts may allow for more specific therapeutic interventions to strengthen the alliance.

Assessment of therapeutic alliance

Although the causal direction of this relationship still requires clarification, preliminary evidence suggests that alliance improves over the course of treatment and this ultimately has an impact on how well people do in treatment and their subsequent success with regard to productive activities and employment. Although several mediating and moderating variables in the alliance–employment relationship have been proposed, these have not been well established. However, there is sufficient evidence to suggest that formally assessing and monitoring the development of the therapeutic alliance over treatment may be useful. This would allow clinicians to check for discrepancies in client, family and/or their own perceptions of the alliance over time. Where there are discrepancies or where views appear to be diverging over time, specific strategies can be implemented. For example, if Client = Family < Therapist, this suggests that the client and family both think the alliance is not as strong as does the therapist. Thus, the therapist may need to rethink his or her views of how things are going and work with both the client and the family to clarify why view of the alliance is weaker. This allows the therapist to review the various elements of the alliance to determine whether it is the bond or a lack of clarity and agreement about goals and tasks in treatment. If the following discrepancy was present, Client < Family = Therapist, then it may be that clarification with the client is needed and the family's congruent views of the alliance with the therapist may mean that they can be helpful in this process. We would argue that measures of alliance should be taken on multiple occasions throughout the course of counselling in order to monitor the development of alliance from multiple perspectives. There are several measures that are likely to have utility in practice.

Probably the two most widely used measures are the WAI (Horvath & Greenberg, 1989) and the CALPAS (Marmar et al., 1989). Both measures have client-, therapist- and observer-rated versions. The WAI has 36 items rated on a 7-point Likert-type scale with subscales that assess bond, task and goals. There is also a shorter 12-item version (Tracey & Kokotovic, 1989). The CALPAS has 30 items and factor analysis has confirmed four factors although the questions are described as mostly reflecting 'purposive mutual work' between the patient and the therapist (Elvins & Green, 2008). A recent review indicated that both were 'well triangulated' with other measures and had good validity data (see Elvins & Green, 2008).

These scales have been adopted from psychotherapy research, and it has been argued that there are important differences between psychotherapy contexts and psychiatric settings that work with individuals with severe and enduring mental illnesses such as schizophrenia (e.g. Elvins & Green, 2008; Priebe & McCabe, 2006). This led to the development of the Scale for the Assessment of Therapeutic Relationships (STAR; McGuire-Snieckus et al., 2007), which focuses on goal and bond aspects of the alliance for people with severe mental illnesses in community mental health settings. The measure comprises 12 items and has both client and clinician scales, but no observer version. However, it is a relatively new measure with limited validity data so far. It is contended that measures specific to these problems and contexts are needed because clients with psychosis have unique symptoms that may affect the therapeutic relationship. For example, it has been argued that clients with psychosis may be more difficult to engage and specific skills to improve communication may be needed (Priebe & McCabe, 2006). Similarly, we have argued that there is a need to emphasise strengths and hope, given that prior life and treatment experiences have often been discouraging for people with long-term, recurring mental illness.

In some studies of alliance in relation to vocational outcomes, family perceptions of the individual patient and therapist relationship were also taken using the CALPAS (e.g. Sherer et al., 2007). Although there are family therapy alliance scales available (e.g. Friedlander et al., 2006) in the context of vocational rehabilitation counselling, these are not likely to be used unless the family is involved in therapy.

Attributes and skills to improve the therapeutic alliance

Ackerman and Hilsenroth (2003) conducted a qualitative review of therapist characteristics (11 studies) and in session activities (16 studies) that were associated with improved therapeutic alliance across a wide range of psychotherapy approaches and settings. Therapist attributes that were found to be related to positive alliance included conveying a sense of being trustworthy, experienced, honest, flexible respectful, confident, interested, alert, friendly, warm and open. It was proposed that these attributes lead to a stronger alliance, which in turn improves outcome. The process was described as 'A benevolent connection between the patient and therapist helps create a warm, accepting, and supportive therapeutic climate that may increase the opportunity for greater patient change' (Ackerman & Hilsenroth, 2003, p. 7). It was further suggested that the client's belief that the treatment relationship is a collaborative effort with the therapist in turn leads to greater investment in the process.

The technique factors found to contribute positively to alliance were exploration, depth, reflection, supportive, active, affirming and conveying understanding. In addition, alliance was related to noting past therapy success, how much they attended to the patient's experience and facilitated expression of affect (Ackerman & Hilsenroth, 2003). The amount of interpretive technique used by therapists was also found to be related to alliance in two studies, but this may be of less utility in vocational rehabilitation contexts. As can be seen, many of these attributes and skills are closely linked to empathy (e.g. warmth and understanding) and other components of the therapeutic relationship proposed by Rogers (1957). Ackerman and Hilsenroth observed that many of the therapist attribute and technique factors associated with positive alliance were also useful in the identification and repair of ruptures to the alliance.

Managing difficulties in the alliance: strains and ruptures

The importance of managing the alliance should not be overlooked. As relationships in general require work to keep them healthy and functional, so too the working alliance is prone to setbacks and challenging periods. There are numerous factors and events that can contribute to a strain in the alliance, or more seriously what is known as an alliance rupture. Signs of problems emerging in the alliance may vary from one or both parties losing motivation through to significant interpersonal conflict. Safran and colleagues suggest that alliance strains and ruptures are common and perhaps should be expected, but if managed well can represent potent change events (e.g. Safran et al., 1990; Safran & Muran, 1996).

It is important to bear in mind that the working relationship (alliance) is not just about being supportive and agreeing upon goals and tasks. It is embedded within the broader landscape of human experience and relationship dimensions (e.g. transference, authentic person-to-person relationship, modelling). This being the case, many of the factors that influence the establishment of, and fluctuations in, the alliance often emanate from ongoing, perhaps unresolved, interpersonal patterns and existential factors (e.g. identity, safety, personal power, place in the world). Although the working relationship within the context of vocational rehabilitation may not aim to address these contextual factors directly, it is a mistake to fail to utilise some basic principles and strategies to keep the person moving forward, supported by an effective alliance. It is also a mistake for workers to fail to address the part they may play in impeding the establishment of a working alliance and/or contributing to alliance strains and ruptures.

Repeating relationship patterns

Each of us has developed patterns of relating associated with our life experiences. The alliance is influenced by the quality of both current and past interpersonal relationships, and the client's relationship style has an effect on therapeutic expectations from both client and worker (Hersoug et al., 2002). For example, clients with an 'under-involved' interpersonal style tend to have poorer alliance and treatment outcomes (Hardy et al., 2001). However, it is not the client's relationship patterns/style alone that explains these poorer outcomes. Rather, difficult client relational style is more likely to elicit negative responses from the worker (Klee et al., 1990). In the under-involved example, the worker may conclude that the client is unmotivated and decide to put more of his or her energy into working with clients who may indicate greater desire for her or his support. Furthermore, the worker's relationship style can similarly elicit positive or negative responses from the client. For example, under-involved workers may demotivate clients, and a paternalistic relationship pattern may elicit a submissive or resistant response from the client. Worker gender differences have also been noted when working with people with psychosis problems and high-relapse-risk clients. Specifically, male workers may act like under-involved fathers and show little commitment to these clients and perhaps express criticism of these clients, while female workers may feel rejected and seek more connection (Stark, 1994; Stark et al., 1992; Stark & Siol, 1994). As found in 'expressed emotion' research, these patterns of relating can have negative impacts on client progress (e.g. Ball et al., 1992; Van Humbeeck et al., 2001).

Working with strains or ruptures in the alliance

Strains in the alliance can be viewed as motivational fluctuations related to the type of interactions occurring between the worker and the client. Although strains or mild tensions are parts of most relationships from time to time, if unchecked these strains could develop into more severe relationship ruptures. Alliance 'ruptures' usually indicate that the client (and/or perhaps the worker) is at best ambivalent about wanting to continue working with this person, or worse is actively seeking ways to terminate the relationship either confrontationally or through emotional and/or physical withdrawal (Safran et al., 1990; Safran & Muran, 1996). Typical features of alliance ruptures are common; interactional phenomenon; consist of both client and worker contributions; and vary in intensity, duration and frequency (Safran & Muran, 1996).

The measure of a skilled worker is in his or her ability to monitor and subtly intervene in negative fluctuations in the alliance as early as possible without creating more unnecessary strain (Safran et al., 1990). As relational strains and ruptures are associated with the types of perceived interactions that occur between the worker and the client, being prepared to examine these interactions is essential for managing the relationship. However, this requires some judgement in terms of identifying the source of the strain or rupture in a non-attached way. For example, a rupture might be related to the worker drifting into a paternalistic or aloof way of relating to the client, with the client reacting by not attending planned meetings or not following through with planned activities. Alternatively, a rupture might be related to the client having unresolved relationship dynamics from a previous relationship and subconsciously bring this into the current relationship (e.g. the client carrying trauma related to previous breaches of trust). In this case the worker needs to explore the possible triggers for such a rupture and try to help the client stay in the present, dealing with current needs and discerning the present relationship from past relationships. In fact in both cases the way to work towards resolving the rupture is to bring the focus of the interaction back onto the interaction itself and taking responsibility for personal contributions to the rupture.

Safran et al. (1990) suggested six strategies to resolve alliance ruptures:

1. Directly discussing the current relationship dynamics and experiences
2. Working to increase awareness of alliance rupture indicators and a sensitivity to changes in the dynamics of the relationship
3. Tracking your own feelings as a signifier of relational change and also as a method of keeping track of what one might be bringing into the working relationship (e.g. one's own emotional refuse)
4. Taking responsibility for one's own contribution to the rupture
5. Working to understand or empathise with the client's experience
6. Practicing being mindful of the relational dynamics in a non-attached way (i.e. being a participant observer – reflection without being caught in automatic reactions)

For many clients, successfully working through relational strains and ruptures might be novel. It can often be a positive experience for clients to work with a worker who is committed to finding a resolution to the relationship difficulties, rather than declining into criticism or withdrawal. The working through of such strains can reinforce the normality of relationship fluctuations and demonstrate that relationship difficulties can be repaired. It has been shown that clients have better outcomes when workers deal with interpersonal conflict directly (Foreman & Marmar, 1985).

Although some clients may find it difficult to stay with the explorative and at times perhaps confrontational aspects of resolving ruptures, the creation of safe physical and psychological spaces to do the work is important. Easing forward initially by gentle probing and clarification rather than going directly to the immediate interpersonal dynamics might help with the re-establishment of safety, the holding frame within which the more difficult work can be done. An example of this might be a gentle reflection or sharing an observation about the changes in the interaction during the sessions (e.g. 'maybe it is just me but you seem to have less to say in our sessions lately'). Further probes might aim to clarify current and recent thoughts and feelings and other life events and experiences in the person's life that could be impacting upon the working relationship. A gentle way of exploring the relationship and examining one's own potential contribution to the strain or rupture can take the form of a reflective self-disclosure (e.g. 'I'm wondering if I may have disappointed you by something I said or did, or didn't say or do. I've been thinking that not being able to get into the course you wanted two weeks ago would have been quite a big deal for you and I don't think I really let you know that I recognised your disappointment with this.'). The client's feelings about the working relationship might also be assessed by exploring how he or she is feeling about working together at the moment, the progress that is being made, what he or she thinks might help improve things, and so on. This line of questioning can also help reinforce the collaborative nature of the relationship and help the client reclaim some of his or her personal power, the loss of which may have been a contributor to the strain or rupture.

Conclusions

There is considerable research in the broad area of psychosocial interventions for mental health problems that indicate a strong therapeutic alliance independently contributes to improved treatment outcomes. There is growing evidence that these effects are also present and important to vocational rehabilitation outcomes. At present it is unclear whether specific strategies that strengthen alliance are necessary for working with individuals who have severe mental illnesses such as schizophrenia, or whether there are specific strategies that are more important in vocational rehabilitation contexts. Thus, the general characteristics and guidelines for assessing, establishing and maintaining a good quality therapeutic alliance are applicable. In addition, a strengths approach that emphasises hopefulness, establishment of a vision for the future, along with specific goals and tasks to achieve this vision is recommended.

References

Ackerman, S.J., & Hilsenroth, M.J. (2003). A review of therapist characteristics and techniques positively impacting the therapeutic alliance. *Clinical Psychology Review*, 23, 1–33.

Ball, R.A., Moore, E., & Kuipers, L. (1992). Expressed emotion in community care staff: a comparison of patient outcome in a nine month follow-up of two hostels. *Social Psychiatry and Psychiatric Epidemiology*, 27, 35–39.

Baumeister, R.F., Bratslavsky, E., Finkenauer, C. & Vohs, K.D. (2001). Bad is stronger than good. *Review of General Psychology*, 5, 323–370.

Bordin, E.S. (1979). The generalizability of the psychoanalytic concept of the working alliance. *Psychotherapy: Theory, Research and Practice*, 16, 252–260.

Bordin, E.S. (1994). Theory and research on the therapeutic working alliance: new directions. In: Horvath, A.O., & Greenberg, L.S. (eds) *The Working Alliance: Theory, Research, and Practice*. New York: Wiley, pp. 13–37.

Bryson, G.J., Bell, M.D., Lysaker, P.H., & Zito, W. (1997). The Work Behavior Inventory: a scale for the assessment of work behavior for people with severe mental illness. *Psychiatric Rehabilitation Journal*, 20, 47–55.

Clarke, S.P., Oades, L., Crowe, T., & Deane, F.P. (2006). Collaborative goal technology: theory and practice. *Psychiatric Rehabilitation Journal, 30*, 129–136.

Couture, S.M., Roberts, M.D.L., Penn, D.L., Cather, C., Otto, M.W., & Goff, D. (2006). Do baseline client characteristics predict the therapeutic alliance in the treatment of schizophrenia? *Journal of Nervous and Mental Disease, 194*, 10–14.

Crowe, T.P., Deane, F.P., Oades, L.G., Caputi, P., & Morland, K.G. (2006). Effectiveness of a collaborative recovery training program in Australia in promoting positive views about recovery. *Psychiatric Services, 57*, 1497–1500.

Davis, L.W., & Lysaker, P.H. (2007). Therapeutic alliance and improvements in work performance over time in patients with schizophrenia. *Journal of Nervous and Mental Disease, 195*, 353–357.

Donnell, C.M., Strauser, D.R., & Lustig, D.C. (2004). The working alliance: rehabilitation outcomes for persons with severe mental illness. *Journal of Rehabilitation, 70*, 12–18.

Duan, C., & Hill, C.E. (1996). The current state of empathy research. *Journal of Counseling Psychology, 43*, 261–274.

Elvins, R., & Green, J. (2008). The conceptualization and measurement of therapeutic alliance: an empirical review. *Clinical Psychology Review, 28*, 1167–1187.

Foreman, S.A., & Marmar, C.R. (1985). Therapist actions that address initially poor therapeutic alliances in psychotherapy. *American Journal of Psychiatry, 142*, 922–926.

Frank, A.F. & Gunderson, J.G. (1990). The role of therapeutic alliance in the treatment of schizophrenia: relationship to course and outcome. *Archives of General Psychiatry, 47*, 228–236.

Friedlander, M.L., Horvath, A.O., Cabero, A., Escudero, V., Heatherington, L., & Martens, M.P. (2006). System for observing family therapy alliances: a tool for research and practice. *Journal of Counseling Psychology, 53*, 214–224.

Gaston, L. (1990). The concept of the alliance and its role in psychotherapy: theoretical and empirical considerations. *Psychotherapy, 27*, 143–153.

Gaston, L., & Marmar, C.R. (1994). The California Psychotherapy Alliance Scales. In: Horvath, A.O., & Greenbert, L.S. (eds) *The Working Alliance: Theory, Research and Practice*. New York: Wiley, pp. 85–108.

Gehrs, M., & Goering, P. (1994). The relationship between the working alliance and rehabilitation outcomes of schizophrenia. *Psychosocial Rehabilitation Journal, 18*, 43–54.

Hardy, G.E., Cahill, J., Shapiro, D.A., Barkham, M., Rees, A., & Macaskill, N. (2001). Client interpersonal and cognitive styles as predictors of response to time-limited cognitive therapy for depression. *Journal of Consulting and Clinical Psychology, 69*, 841–845.

Hersoug, A.G., Monsen, J.T., Havik, O.E., & Hoglend, P. (2002). Quality of early working alliance in psychotherapy: diagnoses, relationship and intrapsychic variables as predictors. *Psychotherapy & Psychosomatics, 71*, 18–27.

Horvath, A.O., & Greenberg, L.S. (1989). Development and validation of the Working Alliance Inventory. *Journal of Counseling Psychology, 36*, 223–233.

Howgego, I.M., Yellowlees, P., Owen, C., Meldrum, L., & Dark, F. (2003). The therapeutic alliance: the key to effective patient outcome? A descriptive review of the evidence in community mental health case management. *Australian and New Zealand Journal of Psychiatry, 37*, 169–183.

Klee, M.R., Abeles, N., & Muller, R.T. (1990). Therapeutic alliance: early indicators, course, and outcome. *Psychotherapy, 27*, 166–174.

Linley, P.A., & Harrington, S. (2006a). Playing to your strengths. *The Psychologist, 19*, 86–89.

Linley, P.A., & Harrington, S. (2006b). Strengths coaching: a potential-guided approach to coaching psychology *International Coaching Psychology Review*, *1*, 37–48.

Lustig, D.C., Strauser, D.R., Rice, N.W., & Rucker, T.F (2002). The relationship between working alliance and rehabilitation outcomes. *Rehabilitation Counseling Bulletin*, *46*, 25–33.

Lustig, D.C., Strauser, D.R., Weems, G.H., Donnell, C.M., & Smith, L.D. (2003). Traumatic brain injury and rehabilitation outcomes: does the working alliance make a difference? *Journal of Applied Rehabilitation Counseling*, *34*, 30–37.

Marmar, C.R., Weiss, D.S., & Gaston, L. (1989). Toward the validation of the California Therapeutic Alliance Rating System. *Psychological Assessment*, *1*, 46–52.

Martin, D.J., Garske, J.P., & Davis, M.K. (2000). Relation of the therapeutic alliance with outcome and other variables: a meta-analytic review. *Journal of Consulting and Clinical Psychology*, *68*, 438–450.

McCabe, R. & Priebe, S. (2004). The therapeutic relationship in the treatment of severe mental illness: a review of methods and findings. *International Journal of Social Psychiatry*, *50*, 196–204.

McGuire-Snieckus, R., McCabe, R., Catty, J., Hanson, L., & Priebe, S. (2007). A new scale to assess the therapeutic relationship in community mental health: STAR. *Psychological Medicine*, *37*, 85–95.

Oades, L.G., Deane, F.P., Crowe, T.P, Lambert, W.G., Kavanagh, D., & Lloyd, C. (2005). Collaborative recovery: an integrative model for working with individuals that experience chronic and recurring mental illness. *Australasian Psychiatry*, *13*, 279–284.

Priebe, S., & McCabe, R. (2006). The therapeutic relationship in psychiatric settings. *Acta Psychiatrica Sadndinavica*, *113* (Suppl. 429), 69–72.

Rogers, C.R. (1957). The necessary and sufficient conditions of therapeutic personality change. *Journal of Consulting Psychology*, *21*, 95–103.

Safran, J.D., Crocker, P., McMain, S., & Murray, P. (1990). Therapeutic alliance rupture as a therapy event for empirical investigation. *Psychotherapy*, *27*, 154–165.

Safran, J.D., & Muran, J.C. (1996). The resolution of ruptures in the therapeutic alliance. *Journal of Consulting and Clinical Psychology*, *64*, 447–458.

Schonberger, M., Humle, F., & Teasdale, T.W. (2006a). The development of the therapeutic working alliance, patients' awareness and their compliance during the process of brain injury rehabilitation. *Brain Injury*, *20*, 445–454.

Schonberger, M., Humle, F., Zeeman, P., & Teasdale, T.W., (2006b). Working alliance and patient compliance in brain injury rehabilitation and their relation to psychosocial outcome. *Neuropsychological Rehabilitation*, *16*, 298–314.

Sherer, M., Evans, C.C., Leverenz, J., Stouter, J., Irby, J.W., Jr., Lee, J.E., & Yablon, S.A. (2007). Therapeutic alliance in post-acute brain injury rehabilitation: predictors of strength of alliance and impact of alliance on outcome. *Brain Injury*, *21*, 663–672.

Stark, F.M. (1994). The therapist–patient relationship with schizophrenic patients. *Behaviour Change*, *11*, 234–241.

Stark, F.M., Lewandowski, L., & Buchkremer, G. (1992). Therapist–patient relationship as a predictor of the course of schizophrenic illness. *European Psychiatrist*, *7*, 161–169.

Stark, F.M., & Siol, T. (1994). Expressed emotion in the therapeutic relationship with schizophrenic patients. *European Psychiatrist*, *9*, 299–303.

Svensson, B., & Hansson, L. (1999). Therapeutic alliance in cognitive therapy for schizophrenic and other long-term mentally ill patient: development and relationship to outcome in an in-patient treatment programme. *Acta Psychiatrica Scandinavica, 99,* 281–287.

Todd, J., & Bohart, A.C. (1994). *Foundations of Clinical and Counselling Psychology,* 2nd edn. New York: Harper Collins.

Tracey, T.J., & Kokotovic, A.M. (1989). Factor structure of the Working Alliance Inventory. *Psychological Assessment, 1,* 207–210.

Van Humbeeck, G., Van Audenhove, C., Pieters, G., De Hert, M., Storms, G., Vertommen, H., Peuskens, J., & Heyrman, J. (2001). Expressed emotion in staff–patient relationships: the professionals' and residents' perspectives. *Social Psychiatry and Psychiatric Epidemiology, 36,* 486–492.

Chapter 8

THE IMPORTANCE OF VOCATION IN RECOVERY FOR YOUNG PEOPLE WITH MENTAL ILLNESS

Chris Lloyd and Geoff Waghorn

Chapter overview

Young people with mental illness are particularly disadvantaged when it comes to participating in vocational training, higher education, or seeking and maintaining employment. A review of the literature reveals that this is due to a number of factors including low expectations by health professionals, stigma and discrimination, symptomatology and lack of clear responsibility for promoting vocational and social outcomes. A useful approach for practitioners to use is a recovery framework combining evidence-based employment and education assistance with mental health care, provided in parallel with brief vocational counselling, illness management skills, training in stigma countering and disclosure strategies, context-specific social skills and skills in social network development. It is concluded that there is an urgent need to link evidence-based vocational practices with quality mental health care in order to restore hope among young people of ever realising their vocational goals and once again feeling included as valued members of society.

Introduction

All community members have the right to work in suitable conditions, which reflect equity, security, human dignity and respect. Work is important to the mental health and well-being of individuals through providing opportunities to develop self-efficacy and self-esteem, key elements in Maslow's (1943) hierarchy of human needs. It is an aspect of life that provides economic security, valued personal roles, social identity and opportunities for individuals to meaningfully contribute to their local community. Benefits associated with work include structuring time and routine, social contact, collective effort and purpose, social identity and status, personal achievement, and regular activity and involvement (Boardman et al., 2003; Harnois & Gabriel, 2000). Access to meaningful work facilitates economic and social participation in society. Opportunities for workforce participation, which contribute to a sense of social connectedness, are considered critical to the mental health and well-being of individuals, organizations, communities and nations (Morrow et al., 2002).

Continuing experiences of social disadvantage can have significant effects on mental health and well-being (Morrow et al., 2002). People with mental illness are among the most disadvantaged groups in society and can face lifelong exclusion from the workplace, often experiencing difficulties in achieving the basic right to work (Harnois & Gabriel, 2000). People with mental illness are sensitive to the negative health effects of unemployment and the associated loss of structure, purpose, roles and diminished sense of personal identity (Boardman et al., 2003). Despite the negative implications of mental illness for employment, work can be essential for maintaining mental health and well-being and for promoting recovery from mental illness. Work is also linked to opportunities for social inclusion in the wider community and provides an important means by which people with mental illness can actively participate in society.

The UK-based Social Exclusion Unit has identified some reasons why mental illness leads to and reinforces social exclusion. These include (1) stigma and discrimination, (2) low expectations by mental health practitioners, (3) lack of clear responsibility for promoting vocational and social outcomes and (4) barriers to engaging in the community and with accessing basic services (ODPM, 2004). To reduce social exclusion, people with mental illness need opportunities to participate in usual life activities and common experiences available in their local community (Corrigan, 2003). Participation in mainstream work, training and education is, therefore, important for providing the everyday socially valued roles necessary for enhancing the social integration and economic participation of people with mental illness.

This chapter examines:

- Barriers to employment among young people with mental illness
- Early intervention and vocational assistance
- Recovery concepts
- The importance of work in recovery
- Steps to facilitate vocational recovery

Literature review

Barriers to employment

Although the majority of people with mental illness would like to work, they are confronted by a challenging number of internal, external and systemic barriers, which impede their employment opportunities and prospects. Recent Australian studies (see Table 8.1) have found extensive non-participation in the labour force among all categories of mental illness, including anxiety disorders. Hence, people with all diagnostic categories of mental illness could benefit from greater participation in effective educational and vocational services.

Table 8.1 Labour force activity by Australians with mental illness aged 15–64 years in 1998.

Persons aged 15–64 years	Not in the labour force (%)	Looking for work (%)	Employed part-time or full-time (%)	Source
Healthy Australians (no long-term health conditions or disability)	19.9	6.3	73.8	ABS (1999) and Waghorn et al., (2004a)
Anxiety disorders (*ICD-10*)	47.1	7.5	45.4	ABS 1999) and Waghorn et al. (2004a); Waghorn and Chant (2005)
Depression (*ICD-10* excluding post natal)	56.4	7.4	36.2	ABS (1999) and Waghorn and Chant (2005)
Bipolar affective disorder (*DSM-III-R*) most with psychotic features	61.8	4.5	28.0	Jablensky et al. (1999) and Waghorn et al. (2007b)
Psychotic disorders (*DSM-III-R*)	75.2	3.7	21.1	Jablensky et al. (1999) and Waghorn et al. (2002)
Schizophrenia (*DSM-III-R*)	80.7	3.0	16.3	Jablensky et al. (1999) and Waghorn et al. (2003)

ICD-10, International Statistical Classification of Diseases and Related Health Problems 10th Revision; DSM-III-R, Diagnostic and Statistical Manual of Mental Disorders, Revised Third Edition.

Mallick et al. (1998) found that financial resources, employment resources and vocational skills presented the greatest barriers to community integration. Financial resources included money to meet financial obligations such as rent, food and other daily expenses. Employment resources were described as employment opportunities and available resources to obtain and maintain employment. Vocational skills included the ability to perform interpersonal and work-related activities required in a job such as following instructions willingly, working with others to perform a group task, completing tasks quickly and accurately, and complying with occupational health and safety regulations in the workplace.

Three types of barriers to employment specific to mental illness have been identified (Rutman, 1994; Waghorn & Lloyd, 2005). These are (1) the impact of mental illness on the person, (2) external barriers such as the nature of the labour market and the availability of suitable employment assistance and (3) other systemic barriers to employment.

The impact of mental illness on the person as a barrier to employment

Employment barriers result directly from the cognitive, positive, negative and disorganised symptoms of psychosis, from side effects of antipsychotic, mood stabilising and antidepressant medications and from subsequent impairments to social skills, sense of self, personal confidence and self-efficacy (Anthony, 1994; Rutman, 1994). Additional barriers to employment can result from the disruptive episodic nature of the disorders and from the impact on self-esteem of any past negative experiences of stigma and unfair discrimination. Furthermore, the timing of illness onset can disrupt formal education and training, impede school-to-work transitions and damage the early stages of career path formation and the acquisition of work values, work ethics and core work skills. Examples of how mental illness causes barriers to employment and how these can be overcome by appropriate interventions are shown in Table 8.2.

Mental illness can produce cognitive, perceptual, affective and interpersonal deficits, each of which may contribute to employment barriers (Rutman, 1994). Of these, the cognitive deficits have more consistent association with unemployment (McGurk et al., 2003; McGurk & Mueser, 2003; Tsang et al., 2000), reduced job tenure (Gold et al., 2002) and poor work performance (Mueser et al., 2001). Cognitive deficits can include problems with attention, sustained attention, memory and executive functioning (Lewis, 2004). In addition, deficits in social cognition (Vauth et al., 2004) are associated with impaired work-related social skills and may underlie the impaired social competence, which influences vocational outcomes (Tsang et al., 2000; Tsang & Pearson, 1996).

Other internal barriers to achieving vocational goals include unpredictable sleeping patterns, fear of failure, fear of relapse, lack of confidence in vocational abilities, difficulties with concentration and fear of resuming work after years of unemployment (Corrigan, 2003; Provencher et al., 2002). In addition, subjective experiences perceived to impact on work functioning (Waghorn et al., 2005a) and self-efficacy for specific core work activities (Waghorn et al., 2005b) have recently been found associated with current vocational status.

The nature of the labour market as a barrier to employment

Educational attainment is a consistent predictor of obtaining employment in the Australian labour market (Waghorn et al., 2003, 2004a). However, most people with mental illness work part-time and few manage both formal study

Table 8.2 Examples of common barriers to employment among people with mental illness.

Type of barrier	Example of barriers	Impact on career paths	Type of interventions needed	Example of interventions
The direct impact of mental illness on the person	Cognitive, positive, negative and disorganised symptoms are often associated with severe mental illness	The typical age of onset at 10–30 years means that secondary and higher education are often disrupted. Suitable education and career paths may not form or may be permanently disrupted	Evidence-based mental health treatment and community based care	Assertive community treatment and care using a strengths-based approach. Help with independent living and setting personal recovery goals
			Support and education for families and carers	Education and support for families through the timely provision of information about mental illness, treatments and the availability of other services and supports in the community
			Evidence-based open employment or evidence-based vocational rehabilitation	The Drake–Becker Individual Placement and Support model of open employment

(Continued)

Table 8.2 (Continued)

Type of barrier	Example of barriers	Impact on career paths	Type of interventions needed	Example of interventions
			Evidence-based supported education to enable participation in accredited vocational training and higher education	Group-based or individual, on or off campus support, to choose a study program, enrol and continue enrolment until course completion
The nature of the labour market and the availability of suitable assistance	Some industries and jobs have only full-time opportunities, require shift work, use overtime extensively or do not offer flexible hours of attendance	Career goals formed prior to becoming ill will have to be revised according to the requirements of particular industries and employers, and according to the feasibility of managing mental health issues in different work settings	Evidence-based open employment and evidence-based vocational rehabilitation	Career counselling, rapid commencement of job searching and job sampling to help the person test their job preferences, and establish limits to the hours of attendance they can sustain at work
	The fluctuating nature of mental illness means that ongoing assistance is needed to maintain employment. Not all vocational services provided time unlimited support	The non-availability of time-unlimited support can lead to premature job loss through problems arising at work which are not easily solved by the person with a mental illness without help	Ongoing time unlimited support, behind the scenes or on-site as required	The employment specialist meets with the worker on a regular basis away from the workplace to discuss work performance and relevant issues emerging or likely to emerge in the workplace

				The employment specialist identifies a work performance issue and a form of assistance or an accommodation to address it Arrangements are made to discuss the problem and its possible solution with the supervisor
Forms of stigma	Some employers are unwilling to employ people with a mental illness. This can be due to low mental health literacy or due to employers being unaware of how a particular mental disorder can be successfully accommodated in their workplace	Rejection by such employers can erode self-esteem and self-efficacy for employment Negative career experiences can disrupt hope of one day restoring a suitable career path	Stigma countering and disclosure strategies can be planned in advance	At job entry, information can be provided to counter stigma and inform the employer about how the mental health condition restricts the hours that can be worked and the type of tasks that are most suitable. The strengths and abilities of the person can be highlighted and strategies for monitoring and maintaining work performance can be discussed

(Continued)

121

Table 8.2 (*Continued*)

Type of barrier	Example of barriers	Impact on career paths	Type of interventions needed	Example of interventions
	Some health professionals do not really believe that people with severe mental illness can work successfully	These health professionals may not disclose this belief to their patients, but may passively enact this belief by not discussing or encouraging participation in vocational rehabilitation	Structural links between treatment services and employment services to facilitate knowledge transfer across both sectors	An employment specialist could be co-located within the community mental health team to regularly discuss opportunities for all clients and to report back on employment outcomes achieved
	Past stigma experiences or negative career experiences can have a lasting impact on people with a serious mental illness	This may cause people with mental illness to be afraid of returning to work or to have low self-efficacy with respect to employment	Focus on the person's job preferences and perceived need for assistance	Assessment of self-stigma, work-related subjective experiences and work-related self-efficacy can be incorporated into the early stages of a vocational assistance programme. These may identify additional avenues for assistance that the person agrees would be helpful and relevant

and employment simultaneously (Waghorn et al., 2004b), a widely used career advancement strategy in the wider community. While little is known about how labour market characteristics constitute barriers to employment, industries which can best accommodate the employment restrictions imposed by mental illness (MacDonald-Wilson et al., 2003; Waghorn et al., 2004a) are likely to provide the most suitable employment opportunities.

Forms of stigma as systemic barriers to employment

Other systemic barriers to employment include community stigma, internalised stigma, stigma among health and vocational professionals, and workplace stigma. Community stigma and unfair discrimination are frequently reported by people with mental illness (World Health Organization, 2001) as adding to the difficulties of obtaining and retaining employment.

This situation is exacerbated by the fact that some people with mental illness endorse stigmatising beliefs about psychiatric disability. This internalised stigma (also known as self-stigma) affects the individual's self-perception and has the potential to impact on the success or failure of employment opportunities (Caltruax, 2003; Corrigan & Watson, 2002). The extent of past stigma experiences and reactions to those experiences can influence personal decisions about whether or not vocational goals are adopted. In addition, past stigma experiences may exert a strong influence on disclosure preferences throughout psychiatric vocational rehabilitation (Waghorn & Lewis, 2002).

Low expectations by mental health professionals

Low vocational expectations by mental health professionals may limit the vocational prospects of people with mental illness. Blankertz and Robinson (1996) believed that health professionals' low vocational expectations of mental health service consumers prevent the majority of people from receiving vocational rehabilitation and supported employment services. Mental health professionals often report that people with mental illness have unrealistic work expectations and goals (Becker et al., 1996). However, direct surveys of consumers have revealed mostly realistic and informed job preferences (Bond, 2004; Mueser et al., 2001). Through examining programmes with low competitive employment outcomes, Gowdy et al. (2003) found that the onus was often placed on individuals to bring up their interests in employment with the mental health service provider. In addition, service providers tended to emphasise prevocational programmes devoted to job preparation, did not pursue rapid assessment and immediate job search or immediate job placement to capitalise on the service users' work motivation, had limited contact with vocational services, had little direct employer contact and provided minimal support to people once they obtained employment. Practitioners need to reclaim employment as part of their core activity and need to involve themselves in more vocational projects (Robdale, 2004).

Early intervention and vocational assistance

The disruptive and disabling effects of first-episode psychotic disorders may be exacerbated by the more general development life phase issues of mid-to-late adolescence and the early adulthood period. Most psychotic disorders first emerge during this critical developmental period in the lifespan and have an adverse effect on social and emotional well-being (Davis et al., 2000). Major developmental challenges of early adult transition include individuating from the family; developing interests, hobbies and skills; discovering and experimenting with sexuality; forming and maintaining relationships; and moving to employment or further study (EPPIC, 2001).

The onset of a severe mental disorder can threaten a sense of self and identity, destabilise valued goals and roles, and degrade social status. Untreated psychosis can have severe effects on young people across social, psychological and biological domains (EPPIC, 2001). A study conducted by Gould et al. (2005) found that young people identified the loss of self and life dreams as key issues. The symptoms of psychosis appearing in adolescence are often the forerunners for what may be lifelong problems in mental health and social well-being (Davis et al., 2000), and profound and lasting changes to psychosocial circumstances. Among the most deleterious and long-lasting of these is the disruption to educational and vocational trajectories, often resulting in long-term unemployment, underemployment or unrealised career goals and educational potential.

Early intervention is seen as having the potential to produce better outcomes for people with psychotic disorders. Effective early intervention offers the hope of restoring normal social and psychological development (National Early Psychosis Project Clinical Guidelines Working Party, 1998). The goals of early intervention can and ought to include reductions in disruption to the family, disruption to employment or education, the need for inpatient care, the need for high-dose antipsychotic medication, the risk of relapse, the risk of suicide and the total cost of treatment (EPPIC, 2001). Gould et al. (2005) suggested that it is important for practitioners to provide incremental opportunities for young people to be involved in occupations that are meaningful in order to remake the link between occupation and normalcy.

Supported education

Evidence-based supported education for people with mental illness is not widely available, even though the evidence suggests that supported education ought to be a standard component of community mental health care (Waghorn et al.,

2004b). Returning to education can restore disrupted education and may be essential to establish or restore career paths. Many young people with mental illness can return to education with appropriate assistance and often formulate career plans during these years (Mowbray et al., 1999). Returning to education can be a better long-term strategy than entry-level employment and may increase career prospects by adding skilled work with more status, responsibility and financial benefits. In addition, supported education can provide access to a stigma-free identity as students rather than as mental health patients (Waghorn et al., 2004b).

Supported education typically takes a rehabilitation approach by providing assistance, preparation and supports to people wishing to pursue secondary or post-secondary education and vocational training (Mowbray & Megivern, 1999). It has also been suggested that supported education can improve the employment outcomes of people with mental illness (Mowbray & Megivern 1999). This important link is supported by Waghorn et al. (2003), who found a positive association between educational attainment and both current and durable employment in a nationally representative sample of people with schizophrenia. Evidence-based practices such as supported employment (Bond, 2004; Shankar, 2005) and supported education (Waghorn et al., 2004b) are considered critical for the community reintegration of people with severe mental illness (Bond et al., 2004).

The need for individualised assistance to maintain employment or education

Job retention is a major challenge for people with mental illness (Xie et al., 1997). There is consistent evidence that ongoing support strategies improve job retention (Bond, 2004). Ongoing support provided by practitioners can take various forms and may include on-site job coaching, regular phone calls to employers to monitor work performance and the need for further workplace accommodations. Support may include job coaching behind the scenes, anticipating and troubleshooting any work-related problems that may arise, and, when appropriate, regular visits to the workplace (Gowdy et al., 2003). People with mental illness readily acknowledge employment restrictions including the need for ongoing support (Waghorn et al., 2004a). The support can be tailored to individual preferences and to the needs of the employer. The intensity of the support can vary with the fluctuating nature of many psychiatric disorders and with the emergence of new challenges in the workplace, such as changing duties, co-workers or supervisors (Waghorn & Lewis, 2002).

For people receiving supported education, similarly flexible forms of continuing support are required. Support may include information on enrolment requirements, assistance in obtaining financial aid, stress management, time management, student rights and information about resources and assistance for people with disabilities and health conditions (Davis & Rinaldi, 2004;

Mowbray et al., 1999). Students also benefit from information on support groups available, choosing a field of study, more effective study habits, choosing a job and scheduling classes (Mowbray et al., 2001). Both education and employment service providers need to be highly accessible and willing to operate by assisting people in their home, workplace or educational facility (Corrigan, 2003; Davis & Rinaldi, 2004).

The need to support and educate employers

Ongoing support to employers may positively influence their hiring decisions. It is essential to educate employers about mental illness, address their fears and ignorance, and ensure that they feel supported in their role of managing employees with mental illness (Shankar, 2005; Shankar & Collyer, 2003). This is best approached by providing a workplace education programme rather than specifically focusing on individuals. Such a programme could include topics such as mental health in the workplace, managing stress and positive working relationships (Waghorn & Lewis, 2002). In addition, facilitating communication between the employer and the person through routine workplace interactions is likely to help reduce any stigma associated with inaccurate beliefs about mental illness (Waghorn & Lewis, 2002).

Recovery concepts

Recovery is defined as the process of overcoming symptoms, psychiatric disability and social handicap (Rickwood, 2004). It involves a redefinition of the self, the emergence of hope and optimism, empowerment and the establishment of meaningful relationships with others (Resnick et al., 2004). Recovery is oriented towards the reconstruction of meaning and purpose in one's life, the performance of valued social roles, the experience of mental health and well-being, and increasing life satisfaction. It means maximising well-being within the constraints that may be imposed by residual psychiatric symptoms. Best practice incorporates the provision of continuing care, comprising relapse prevention plans and rehabilitation provided within a recovery orientation. The lived experience of people with the mental illness is acknowledged and the goals include maximising their wellness and well-being along with that of their family (Rickwood, 2004).

One of the primary goals of psychiatric rehabilitation is to help people with mental illness recover (Corrigan, 2003). Recovery-focused rehabilitation interventions typically promote the goals of community integration, improved quality of life, personal empowerment and recovery (Casper et al., 2002). Practices that serve these goals and have an underpinning evidence base include individualised supports, consumer choice, skills training, supported employment, supported education, peer support and social network development (Casper et al., 2002). Consumers, however, have not consistently specified access to socially valued roles as a necessary ingredient of definitions of recovery. A recent review by Andresen et al. (2003) of 28 experiential accounts of recovery, consisting of 14 articles written by consumers and 8 qualitative studies, concluded that while a return to expected roles was not considered necessary for recovery, the re-establishment of personal goals, taking personal responsibility and making one's own choices were consistent themes in consumer recovery concepts.

The importance of work in recovery

Having a reason to get out of bed and something meaningful to do during the day is essential for the well-being of people with mental illness. Work has an important role in recovery and many of the general goals of rehabilitation and recovery are best served by addressing the person's vocational aspirations (Corrigan, 2003). The potential importance of work and study to recovery is recognised by Liberman et al. (2002). These researchers developed an operational definition of recovery, which includes a return to work or study as an essential dimension with the added benefit of being capable of objective measurement. The operational criteria have been successfully tested in focus groups composed of clients, family members, practitioners and researchers. The inclusion of socially valued role functioning within an operational definition of recovery was endorsed by all stakeholders.

Vocational activities can contribute to the recovery process in two ways: firstly, through work being perceived as a means of self-empowerment, and secondly, through work promoting a sense of independent identity and self-esteem (Provencher et al., 2002). However, when competitive employment is not a current goal, meaning and purpose can be sought via participation in other contributing roles as a partner, parent or carer, in education, self-development or voluntary work, or through other artistic, social or recreational activities in the community (Waghorn et al., 2007a). Practitioners need to use client-centred assessment in which they determine the individual's abilities, problems, wishes and interests. It is important that they focus on the strengths of the person in order to motivate them to be involved in the intervention by building a programme of intervention on their wishes and interests.

Facilitating vocational recovery

Initiating conversations about work and education

It is important that practitioners initiate conversations about work and education in the early stages of involvement with the service. The availability of suitable employment programmes and supported education programmes can be discussed along with the person's career aspirations (Gowdy et al., 2003).

This is best done using a strengths-based approach, with clear expectations of vocational recovery. Strengths elements include identifying the person's interests, talents, abilities and resources; discussing current roles, responsibilities and mutual expectations of the rehabilitative relationship; and regularly updating details of interests and achievements and resources in the person's own words (Waghorn & Lewis, 2002). People who have not worked for a year or more may fear employment and may under- or overestimate their capabilities. Practitioners may need to discuss any concerns associated with working and assist individuals to overcome their fears through encouragement and supported exposure and through appropriate work-related strategies (Gowdy et al., 2003). For people who need to complete high school or who desire higher education or vocational training, education goals can be explored in relation to longer-term career interests.

Vocational counselling and assessment

Brief forms of vocational assessments and person-centred vocational counselling can be used to narrow the available education and employment options. However, due to the impact of mental illness and the likelihood of career immaturity, extensive assessment of abilities and career interests are not warranted and do not predict outcomes any better than the person's own preferences (Bond, 2004). Practitioners often work with clients in their natural environments where it has been found that clients feel more confident to open up during the doing process (Whitcher & Tse, 2004).

Career counselling can be brief and exploratory and can occur in parallel with more active forms of vocational assistance (e.g. job searching) in order to build on a person's current motivation and job preferences while not delaying attainment of the primary employment goal (Bond, 2004). Waghorn et al. (2007b) suggest using a multidimensional measure of socially valued role functioning in the early stage of vocational assistance. This measure is expected to help individuals in reviewing current role activities and in selecting opportunities within available role options. For instance, a person may express employment interest, yet when asked about other role activities, may reveal an existing ongoing commitment to care for children or an ageing person, an equally important role which may not currently allow sufficient time or energy to be diverted to vocational goals.

Skills training

People who lack sufficient interpersonal skills to get by in the workplace will experience difficulty in achieving their vocational goals. Practitioners utilise strategies that assist people to learn and use social skills that are necessary for some people to take advantage of opportunities in their community. The findings from the study conducted by Mairs and Bradshaw (2004) suggest that life skills training approaches can reduce symptoms.

People need to be able to obtain information about vocational opportunities, inquire about required skills, job openings or course availability, and frequently need to complete application forms (Roder et al., 2001). People also need sufficient social skills for common workplace situations such as asking questions during a job interview, talking with co-workers during breaks, cooperating with co-workers to perform a group task and checking instructions with a supervisor (Waghorn et al., 2007a; Waghorn & Lewis, 2002).

Coping skills can be taught that assist people to address unexpected blocks to the attainment of their goals (Corrigan, 2003). People may experience such problems as rejection of a job application or interpersonal difficulties with co-workers. Strategies utilised by practitioners that can be taught include stress management, relaxation training, work-related communication and problem solving (Roder et al., 2001). Social skills are usually taught in a staged process, which includes being introduced to the skills, role rehearsal, video feedback and homework assignments (Lloyd et al., 2004).

To enable the skills taught to generalise beyond the training context, people need to be able to practice their newly learned skills in a variety of venues away from the treatment setting. Homework activities are important, through requiring people to rehearse the new skills in a setting with different social demands (Corrigan, 2003). The main caveat is that for people with education or employment goals, any prevocational or general rehabilitative training should not delay active vocational assistance (Bond, 2004) and can be focused on the particular employment or educational context the person is seeking (Tsang, 2001; Tsang & Pearson, 1996).

In addition, people may need training and support to access community resources. People require basic resources such as income support, housing, access to transport, and good mental and physical health care, which are critical both to promote positive mental health and to enable people to take up opportunities in the community (Corrigan, 2003; ODPM, 2004). Practitioners are able to explore the ways they can assist people to access community resources (Heasman & Atwal, 2004). People with mental illness often experience financial hardship and may need assistance with budget planning, income support and benefit entitlements, which, if not addressed, could adversely affect vocational motivation (Bond, 2004).

Intersectoral partnerships

It is important that community mental health service staff establish structural links with local disability employment services and educational institutions (Davis & Rinaldi, 2004). According to Davis and Rinaldi (2004), clients attaching a high priority to work and the social inclusion policy agenda highlighted the advantages of the involvement of practitioners in the vocational rehabilitation process. In addition, the most successful services integrate mental health care with employment assistance, an approach which has been shown to outperform brokered arrangements (Bond, 2004). Intersectoral partnerships can also be used to help people explore community opportunities. The incorporation of evidence-based practice within vocational rehabilitation into the community mental health team has led a shift from a purely medical outcome to a social outcome of gaining employment, education or voluntary work (Davis & Rinaldi, 2004).

Network development

People with mental illness usually have small social networks that lack stability and reciprocity in relationships (Heasman & Atwal, 2004; Shankar & Collyer, 2003). The availability of supports can positively influence employment (Shankar & Collyer, 2003) and educational outcomes (Mowbray et al., 2001). Any interventions provided by practitioners can be complemented by interventions that strengthen and support the individual's social network. Social support helps the person meet basic needs for affection and affiliation (Corrigan, 2003) and facilitates a sense of belonging in their community. This can be achieved by increasing people's opportunities for community participation by increasing access to education, volunteering, employment, arts and leisure (Black & Living, 2004; Davis & Rinaldi, 2004; Heasman & Atwal, 2004; ODPM, 2004). Practitioners may work with people who may need assistance to take up activities of interest in mainstream settings in addition to any activities provided by support groups. Supportive social networks can promote a sense of well-being, help develop social confidence and encourage greater access to educational and employment opportunities.

Conclusions

The challenge for practitioners is to find ways to sensibly combine evidence-based practices from the mental health care, early intervention, and the specialised employment and supported education domains. Only then can we offer hope to people with mental illness for attainment of a relatively normal life. Becoming a mentally restored person through clinical treatment and mental health care is neither sufficient nor socially just, because people in full remission without symptoms often fail to return to socially valued roles in the community. People need appropriately intensive and continuing assistance, which aims to restore the secondary disabilities associated with being denied socially valued role opportunities and through having a spoiled social identity. Using a recovery framework, mental health services can make a difference, provided their efforts encompass rather than exclude vocational attainment as a realistic and appropriate goal for people with mental illness.

The main implication for mental health professionals is that the traditional approach of providing community-based mental health treatment and care needs to continue. However, the traditional focus on prevocational skills training, life skills education or general rehabilitative programmes in the mental health setting, unlinked to any systematic efforts to restore vocational functioning, can no longer be justified. In other words, traditional rehabilitation activities must give way to evidence-based practices, especially when people express a preference for employment or a return to formal education. However, once an employment context is identified, or employment or education commences, various forms of skills training (e.g. illness management at work, work-related social skills training) can be productively applied in a particular setting leveraged by the person's vocational motivation and perceptions of relevance.

Acknowledgement

This chapter is reprinted with permission from the *British Journal of Occupational Therapy* (Lloyd, C., & Waghorn, G. (2007). The importance of vocation in recovery for young people with psychiatric disabilities. *British Journal of Occupational Therapy, 70,* 50–59.)

References

Andresen, R., Oades, L., & Caputi, P. (2003). The experience of recovery from schizophrenia: towards an empirically validated stage model. *Australian and New Zealand Journal of Psychiatry, 37,* 586–594.

Anthony, W.A. (1994). Characteristics of people with psychiatric disabilities that are predictive of entry into the rehabilitation process and successful employment. *Psychosocial Rehabilitation Journal, 17,* 3–13.

Australian Bureau of Statistics (ABS, 1999). Survey of disability, ageing, and carers, Australia. Technical paper. Confidentialized unit record file 1998. Canberra: Commonwealth Government.

Becker, D., Drake, R., Farabaugh, A., & Bond, G. (1996). Job preference of clients with severe mental disorders participating in supported employment programs. *Psychiatric Services, 47,* 1223–1226.

Black, W., & Living, R. (2004). Volunteerism as an occupation and its relationship to health and wellbeing. *British Journal of Occupational Therapy, 67,* 526–532.

Blankertz, R., & Robinson, S. (1996). Adding a vocational focus to mental health rehabilitation. *Psychiatric Services, 47,* 1216–1222.

Boardman, J., Grove, B., Perkins, R., & Shepherd, G. (2003). Work and employment for people with psychiatric disabilities. *British Journal of Psychiatry, 182,* 467–468.

Bond, G. (2004). Supported employment: evidence for an evidence-based practice. *Psychiatric Rehabilitation Journal*, *27*, 345–359.

Bond, G., Salyers, M., Rollins, A., Rapp, C., & Zipple, A. (2004). How evidence-based practices contribute to community integration. *Community Mental Health Journal*, *40*, 569–588.

Caltruax, D. (2003). Internalized stigma: a barrier to employment for people with mental illness. *International Journal of Therapy and Rehabilitation*, *10*, 539–543.

Casper, E., Oursler, J., Schmidt, L., & Gill, K. (2002). Measuring practitioners' beliefs, goals, and practices in psychiatric rehabilitation. *Psychiatric Rehabilitation Journal*, *23*, 223–234.

Corrigan, P., & Watson, A.C. (2002). The paradox of self-stigma and mental illness. *Clinical Psychology: Science and Practice*, *9*, 35–53.

Corrigan, P.W. (2003). Beat the stigma: come out of the closet. *Psychiatric Services*, *54*, 1313.

Davis, C., Martin, G., Kosky, R., & O'Hanlon, A. (2000). *Early Intervention in the Mental Health of Young People*. Adelaide: The Australian Early Intervention Network for Mental Health in Young People.

Davis, M., & Rindaldi, M. (2004). Using an evidence-based approach to enable people with mental health problems to gain and retain employment, education and voluntary work. *British Journal of Occupational Therapy*, *67*, 319–322.

EPPIC (2001). *Case Management in Early Psychosis: A Handbook*. Melbourne: EPPIC.

Gold, J.M., Goldberg, R.W., McNary, S.W., Dixon, L.B., & Lehman, A.F. (2002). Cognitive correlates of job tenure among patients with severe mental illness. *American Journal of Psychiatry*, *159*, 1395–1402.

Gould, A., DeSouza, S., & Rebeiro-Gruhl, K.L. (2005). And then I lost that life: a shared narrative of four young men with schizophrenia. *British Journal of Occupational Therapy*, *68*, 467–473.

Gowdy, L., Carlson, L., & Rapp, C. (2003). Practices differentiating high-performing from low-performing supported employment programs. *Psychiatric Rehabilitation Journal*, *26*, 232–239.

Harnois, G., & Gabriel, P. (2000). *Mental Health and Work: Impact, Issues and Good Practices*. Geneva: World Health Organization and International Labour Organisation.

Heasman, D., & Atwal, A. (2004). The Active Advice Pilot Project: leisure enhancement and social inclusion for people with severe mental health problems. *British Journal of Occupational Therapy*, *67*, 511–514.

Jablensky, A., McGrath, J., Herrman, H., Castle, D., Gureje, O., Morgan, V., & Korten, A. (1999). *National Survey of Mental Health and Wellbeing. Report 5. People Living with Psychotic Illness: An Australian Study*. Canberra: Mental Health Branch, Commonwealth Department of Health and Aged Care.

Lewis, R. (2004). Should cognitive deficit be a diagnostic criterion for schizophrenia? *Journal of Psychiatry Neuroscience*, *29*, 102–113.

Liberman, R.P., Kopelowicz, A., Ventura, J., & Gutkind, D. (2002). Operational criteria and factors related to recovery from schizophrenia. *International Review of Psychiatry*, *14*, 256–272.

Lloyd, C., Williams, P.L., & Sullivan, D. (2004). Kick'n'On: helping young males kick back into life. *Australian e-Journal for the Advancement of Mental Health* *3*(2), www.auseinet.com/journal/vol3iss2/lloyd.pdf (accessed 27 December 2008).

Mairs, H., & Bradshaw, T. (2004). Life skills training in schizophrenia. *British Journal of Occupational Therapy*, *67*, 217–224.

Mallick, K., Reeves, R., & Dellario, D. (1998). Barriers to community integration for people with severe and persistent disabilities. *Psychiatric Rehabilitation Journal*, 22, 175–180.

Maslow, A.H. (1943). A theory of human motivation. *Psychological Review*, 50, 370–396.

McGurk, S.R., & Mueser, K.T. (2003). Cognitive functioning and employment in severe mental illness. *Journal of Nervous and Mental Disease*, 191, 789–798.

McGurk, S.R., Mueser, K.T., Harvey, P.D., La Puglia, R., & Marder, J. (2003). Cognitive and symptom predictors of work outcomes for clients with schizophrenia in supported employment. *Psychiatric Services*, 54, 1129–1135.

Morrow, L., Verins, I., & Willis, E. (2002). *Mental Health and Work Issues and Perspectives*. Adelaide, Auseinet: The Australian Network for Promotion, Prevention and Early Intervention for Mental Health.

Mowbray, C., Bybee, D., & Collins, M. (2001). Follow-up client satisfaction in a supported education program. *Psychiatric Rehabilitation Journal*, 24, 237–247.

Mowbray, C., Collins, M., & Bybee, D. (1999). Supported education for individuals with psychiatric disabilities: long-term outcomes from an experimental study. *Social Work Research*, 23, 89–100.

Mowbray, C., & Megivern, D. (1999). Higher education and rehabilitation for people with psychiatric disabilities. *Journal of Rehabilitation*, 65, 31–38.

Mueser, K.T., Becker, D.R., & Wolfe, R.S. (2001). Supported employment, job preferences, job tenure and satisfaction. *Journal of Mental Health*, 10, 411–417.

National Early Psychosis Project Clinical Guidelines Working Party (1998). *Australian Clinical Guidelines for Early Psychosis*. Melbourne: National Early Psychosis Project, University of Melbourne.

Office of the Deputy Prime Minister (ODPM, 2004). *Mental Health and Social Exclusion*. Wetherby, UK: ODPM Publications.

Provencher, H., Gregg, R., Mead, S., & Mueser, K. (2002). The role of work in the recovery of persons with psychiatric disabilities. *Psychiatric Rehabilitation Journal*, 26, 132–144.

Resnick, S.G., Rosenheck, R., & Lehman, A. (2004). An exploratory analysis of correlates of recovery. *Psychiatric Services*, 55, 540–547.

Rickwood, D. (2004). *Pathways of Recovery: Preventing Relapse*. Canberra: Department of Health and Ageing.

Robdale, N. (2004). Vocational rehabilitation: the Enable Employment Retention Scheme, a new approach. *British Journal of Occupational Therapy*, 67, 457–460.

Roder, V., Zorn, P., Muller, D., & Brenner, H. (2001). Improving recreational, residential, and vocational outcomes for patients with schizophrenia. *Psychiatric Services*, 52, 1439–1441.

Rutman, I.D. (1994). How psychiatric disability expresses itself as a barrier to employment. *Psychosocial Rehabilitation Journal*, 17, 15–35.

Shankar, J. (2005). Improving job tenure for people with psychiatric disabilities through ongoing employment support. *Australian e-Journal for the Advancement of Mental Health*, 4(1) www.auseinet.com/jounal/vol4iss1/shankar.pdf (accessed 27 December 2008).

Shankar, J., & Collyer, F. (2003). Vocational rehabilitation of people with mental illness: the need for a broader approach. *Australian e-Journal for the Advancement of Mental Health*, 2(2) www.auseinet.com/journal/vol2iss2/shankar.pdf (accessed 27 December 2008).

Tsang, H., Lam, P., Ng, B., & Leung, O. (2000). Predictors of employment outcome for people with psychiatric disabilities: a review of the literature since the mid 80s. *Journal of Rehabilitation*, 66, 19–31.

Tsang, H.W.H. (2001). Applying social skills training in the context of vocational rehabilitation for people with schizophrenia. *Journal of Nervous and Mental Disease, 189,*
90–98.

Tsang, H.W.H., & Pearson, V. (1996). A conceptual framework for work-related social
skills in psychiatric rehabilitation. *Journal of Rehabilitation, 62,* 61–67.

Vauth, R., Rusch, N., Wirtz, M., & Corrigan, P.W. (2004). Does social cognition influence
the relation between neurocognitive deficits and vocational functioning in schizophrenia?
Psychiatry Research, 128, 155–165.

Waghorn, G., & Chant, D. (2005). Labour force activity by people with depression and anxiety disorders: a population level second order analysis. *Acta Psychiatrica Scandinavica,*
112, 415–424.

Waghorn, G., Chant, D., & Jaeger, J. (2007b). Employment functioning among community
residents with bipolar affective disorder: results from an Australian community survey.
Bipolar Disorders, 9, 166–182.

Waghorn, G., Chant, D., & King, R. (2005a). Work-related subjective experiences among
community residents with schizophrenia or schizoaffective disorder. *Australian and New*
Zealand Journal of Psychiatry, 39, 88–99.

Waghorn, G., Chant, D., & King, R. (2005b). Work-related self-efficacy among community
residents with psychiatric disabilities. *Psychiatric Rehabilitation Journal, 29,* 105–113.

Waghorn, G., Chant, D., & King, R. (2007a). Classifying socially-valued role functioning
among community residents with psychiatric disorders. *American Journal of Psychiatric*
Rehabilitation, 10, 185–221.

Waghorn, G., Chant, D., White, P., & Whiteford, H. (2004a). Delineating disability, labour
force participation and employment restrictions among persons with psychosis. *Acta Psy-*
chiatrica Scandinavica, 109, 279–288.

Waghorn, G., Chant, D., & Whiteford, H. (2002). Clinical and non-clinical predictors of
vocational recovery for Australians with psychotic disorders. *Journal of Rehabilitation,*
68, 40–51.

Waghorn, G., Chant, D., & Whiteford, H. (2003). The strength of self-reported course
of illness in predicting vocational recovery for persons with schizophrenia. *Journal of*
Vocational Rehabilitation, 18, 33–41.

Waghorn, G., & Lewis, S. (2002). Disclosure of psychiatric disabilities in vocational rehabilitation. *Australian Journal of Rehabilitation Counselling, 8,* 67–80.

Waghorn, G., & Lloyd, C. (2005). The employment of people with a mental illness. *Aus-*
tralian e-Journal for the Advancement of Mental Health, 4(2, Suppl.), www.auseinet.com/
journal/vol4iss2suppl/waghornlloyd.pdf (accessed 27 December 2008).

Waghorn, G., Still, M., Chant, D., & Whiteford, H. (2004b). Specialised supported education
for Australians with psychotic disorders. *Australian Journal of Social Issues, 39,* 443–458.

Whitcher, K., & Tse, S. (2004). Counselling skills in occupational therapy: a grounded
theory approach to explain use within mental health in New Zealand. *British Journal of*
Occupational Therapy, 67, 361–368.

World Health Organization (2001). The World Health Report 2001 – Mental Health: New
Understanding, New Hope. Geneva: World Health Organization.

Xie, H., Dain, B.J., Becker, D.R., & Drake, R.E. (1997). Job tenure among people with
severe mental illness. *Rehabilitation Counseling Bulletin, 40,* 230–239.

Chapter 9

EMPLOYMENT AND EARLY PSYCHOSIS

Niall Turner

Chapter overview

People recovering from early psychosis regard returning to work or education as the key in their recovery. While clinicians dedicate time, energy and effort to assist people attain this goal, on many occasions attempts are unsuccessful. In the last decade there has been increased interest in preventing the disability associated with psychosis through early detection and assertive treatment in the first 3–5 years post-onset of psychosis. Vocational interventions are often, but not always, part of this treatment. The individual placement and support model of supported employment has proven effective with people in the early phase of a psychotic condition. However, employment may not always be the most appropriate goal or outcome for a young person recovering from an episode of psychosis; completing education or training may be the priority. Although calls for equal importance be afforded to functional recovery, the investment in evidence-based interventions that have the potential to make this a reality is lacking. This chapter concludes that greater investment and more research is required to find the most appropriate models for assisting people recovering from early psychosis achieve meaningful lives.

Introduction

Paid employment is the common means of achieving adequate economic resources which are essential for people to fully participate in society. Work is considered important enough to warrant articles in the Universal Declaration of Human Rights (1948), the International Covenant on Economic, Social and Cultural Rights (1966) and the African Charter on Human and Peoples' Rights (1981). Furthermore scientific study has borne out the anecdotal evidence of the benefits of work to our health and well-being (Waddell & Burton, 2006).

In societies where employment is the norm, work becomes central to a person's identity, social roles and community status. There is stigma attached to being without work and people can be regarded as being lazy, idle and even wasteful if they reveal they are not working. The majority of people with psychiatric illness, particularly conditions that feature psychosis such as schizophrenia, face this stigma, as successful return to employment or education is uncommon. The stigma attached to being unemployed further compounds the stigma people with psychosis already face as a result of the negative public attitudes towards mental illness.

The impact of psychosis can be devastating for the individual and their family (Clarke & O'Callaghan, 2003). Adolescence and early adulthood are the greatest period of risk for developing psychosis, coinciding with a critical time of occupational development. Employment outcomes for people with schizophrenia are very poor, with as few as 4% of a group of people with schizophrenia employed in a study conducted in the developed world 10 years ago at a time of good employment among the general population (Perkins & Rinaldi, 2002). It is only those with severe learning disabilities who are less likely to be in paid work (Boardman, 2003). Low rates of employment are confined to not just people with enduring schizophrenia but also among people experiencing their first episode of psychosis in part due to delays in receiving effective treatment (Turner et al., 2009).

In an attempt to prevent the development of the secondary disabilities associated with psychosis, an early intervention approach was pioneered in Australia in the early 1990s and has been adopted in nearly 200 mental health services around the globe (McGorry et al., 2007). The key principles of early intervention are to reduce the delays to effective treatment and provide interventions tailored specifically for the early stages of a psychotic condition. Vocational rehabilitation often, but not always, forms part of this treatment.

Supported employment is now proving more successful than previous attempts at vocational rehabilitation (Crowther et al., 2001), particularly when integrated in the mental health service (Cook et al., 2005). Models of vocational rehabilitation for early psychosis have yet to be finalised and as a result there are currently different innovative approaches being developed and trialled. Integrated supported employment models have shown promising results in early psychosis populations (Killackey et al., 2008; Rinaldi et al., 2004). However, the employment needs of young people with psychosis may differ substantially from the needs of more enduring populations where supported employment was developed.

Developing a vocational programme for young people with psychosis presents both opportunities and challenges whether the programme is part of an early intervention service or a generic mental health service. The key to getting a programme up and running is developing a vision of the programme and then achieving widespread 'buy in' from people who will be availing the programme, those who will be potentially referring to the programme and those who will be funding the programme. Subsequently, the key to maintaining support is evaluating the benefits and disseminating the results.

In evaluating vocational interventions, employment is considered a key outcome variable; however, definitions of employment are inconsistent (Marwaha & Johnson, 2004). Binary variables of employed/unemployed or working/not working are often presented, but the method of categorisation is not always provided. The question arises whether full-time students or full-time parents should be considered working or not working/employed or unemployed? Considering those in education as not working may be underestimating their achievement and the achievement of the service that assisted in getting them there.

This chapter examines:

- The early psychosis paradigm
- Getting started in developing a vocational programme for early psychosis
- Establishing the need for vocational programmes for early psychosis
- Vocational programmes for early psychosis with a emerging evidence base
- Real world examples of vocational programmes in early intervention services
- Measuring success of vocational programmes for early psychosis

The early psychosis paradigm

Although over 200 early intervention services have now been established across the world, the early psychosis paradigm is still a relatively new approach to clinicians. Most clinicians have worked in traditional services where the two main paradigms of care for people with psychosis are (1) acute crisis care and (2) rehabilitation. By following these paradigms, the interventions – biological and psychosocial – have traditionally neglected to take into account the phase or age of the illness (Birchwood et al., 1998).

An approach that does not take into account the phase or age of the illness assumes that a 'one size fits all' model is effective; however, the needs of a person in the acute phase of their first episode of psychosis and their subsequent rehabilitative needs are substantially different from those of someone who has a 10-year history of a remitting/relapsing course of schizophrenia.

Also, is it possible that the period immediately after the first onset of psychosis is an opportunity to influence the likely course of the condition? McGorry et al. (1996) outlined a phase-orientated classification of psychosis where a clear distinction is made between the phase of 'early' psychosis – precursors, prodrome and period of first episode of psychosis – and the phase of 'prolonged' psychosis. The 'critical period' outlined by Birchwood et al. (1998) is the intermediate phase between the two. It is during this early phase and critical period that it is proposed the course of the condition can be influenced and the secondary impairments and disabilities associated with psychosis can be prevented. Due to the aggressive development of disability in the first 2–3 years, it is suggested that assertive intervention for this period of time is warranted (Birchwood et al., 1998).

This new phase-orientated classification of psychosis leads to the development of early intervention for psychosis services. These services tailor their approach to the needs of someone who is experiencing early psychosis by providing interventions orientated to younger people provided at the earliest opportunity, usually in a setting separate to those in the 'prolonged' psychosis phase.

A cornerstone of early intervention services is reducing delays to effective treatment, known as duration of untreated psychosis (DUP). Commonly, DUP among those with psychosis is 1–2 years (Marshall et al., 2005). Delays have many adverse consequences, including reduced quality of life (Browne et al., 2000), increased risk of self-harm (Clarke et al., 2006), diminished purpose in life (Turner et al., 2007), higher symptom severity at first presentation (Melle et al., 2004), poorer functioning at first presentation (Melle et al., 2004), worse short-term outcome (Marshall et al., 2005) and medium-term outcome (Whitty et al., 2008). There is also some evidence that delays have a negative impact on employment. Barnes et al. (2000) found that 46% of a group of people with delays of less than the median delay (26 weeks) were still employed or in education compared to 22% of those with long delays. More recently, an Irish study found those unemployed amongst a group of people with psychosis had longer DUP than those employed or those in non-labour force work (students, home maintainer, retired) (Turner et al., 2009). In addition of concern is the impact of initial delays on later occupational functioning. Norman et al. (2007) examined the occupational activity of young people who had used an early intervention for psychosis service 3 years after starting treatment. Occupational activity was measured as the number of weeks in a year in paid employment or attending school. Results show that 28% had full-time occupation throughout the year, of which 73% were in paid employment. Greater full-time occupational activity was associated with better education, higher initial capacity for work (as rated by case managers), better premorbid adjustment, shorter DUP and higher levels of social support, with the latter two having the strongest influence.

Fortunately DUP is malleable; a number of early intervention services have reduced delays. The Canadian service PEPP achieved a 50% reduction from 16 to 8 months (Malla et al., 2003); the TIPS project in Norway reduced DUP from 29 to 6 months in an area where a professional and public education campaign was delivered, whereas the DUP in the control area remained the same (Friis et al., 2005). In Australia the EPPIC service cut delays from 18 to 11 months (McGorry et al., 1996), and in Singapore delays were shortened to 4 months after the introduction of an awareness campaign, a reduction of 8 months from the pre-campaign average DUP of 12 months (Chong et al., 2005).

Some evidence, presented in Table 9.1, has shown that early intervention services, even without specific occupational interventions, can improve

Table 9.1 Improved occupational outcomes.

OPUS trial[a]	LEO service[b]	Soteria Nacka study[c]
The OPUS trial is a randomised control trial of an integrated specialist service for the critical period versus standard treatment. At 1 year those in the 'all psychoses' or 'schizophrenia only' groups receiving integrated treatment were 69 and 41%, respectively, less likely to have no work/not in education in comparison to those in standard treatment.	In a UK randomised control trial of the Lambeth Early Onset service, the 71 people with psychosis receiving the specialised care were 3.4 times more likely to participate in vocational interventions on offer and were 59% more likely to achieve full or partial recovery at 18 months than those receiving standard care ($n = 73$).	In a quasi-experimental evaluation of an early intervention in Sweden, 5-year employment/education outcomes were significantly better amongst those who availed of the 'comprehensive' first episode care in comparison to outpatient care; only 20% (75 to 55%) lost employment in comparison to 43% (63 to 20%) of those in standard outpatient care.

[a] Petersen et al. (2005).
[b] Craig et al. (2004).
[c] Lindgren et al. (2006).

occupational outcomes. However, the International Early Psychosis Association guidelines suggest that specific programmes should be developed to assist those in the early phase of psychosis return to purposeful work.

More recently, a group of clinicians interested in both early psychosis and vocational recovery launched the International First Episode Vocational Recovery statement at the International Early Intervention in Psychosis conference in Melbourne Australia 2008 (The International First Episode Vocational Recovery Group, 2008). Meaningful Lives is an international consensus statement setting out the challenge, the benefits, the principals, goals and processes for occupation recovery to become a reality for people with psychosis. The key principles and goals are presented in Table 9.2; for further information log onto http://www.iris-initiative.org.uk/recovery-and-ordinary-lives/.

Starting out

Developing and implementing a vocational programme for young people with psychosis is not straightforward, as anyone who has done so will testify. Different approaches may be necessary depending on the environment where the programme is being proposed. The setting may be a specialist early intervention

Table 9.2   Key principles and goals.

The key principles are	The goals are to
• All young people have a right to education, training and employment • All young people have the right to citizenship and a basic income to live on • All young people have the right to develop a career that gives meaning to their lives and makes use of their talents • Young people with psychosis should have the same education and vocational opportunities as their peers • No individual should be discriminated against or disadvantaged in relation to their educational and vocational aspirations because they have had a serious mental health difficulty • Educational as well as vocational outcomes should be equally valued and supported in first-episode psychosis	• Combat stigma and discrimination in workplace and education settings • Support young people attain their education, training and employment outcomes • Ensure that functional outcomes are given equal priority to symptomatic recovery • Advocate with funding agencies to appropriately resource evidence-based interventions to address the functional outcomes in relation to education, training and employment • Combat factors that contribute to social exclusion and unfulfilled lives • Encourage professional attitudes that engender hope and optimism that young people with psychosis can lead meaningful lives

for psychosis service, as not all have well-developed vocational programmes, or may be in a generic mental health service where early intervention has yet to be established. Following a planning process like that presented in Box 9.1 can work for either setting.

Establishing the need for the vocational programme

In order to secure the necessary resources to establish a vocational programme in either an early intervention service or a generic service, the requirements for the programme will firstly need to be established and then a convincing argument and proposal put to funding agencies. Some points that can be used to argue for vocational programmes include:

• The importance of work to society
• The importance of work to service users
• The benefits of employment and perils of worklessness

> **Box 9.1   Planning a vocational programme for young people with psychosis**
>
> Establish the need for the programme
> Gain support for a vocational programme among the staff
> Evaluate relevant research including qualitative research of the service user's views
> Develop a vision of the programme based on steps 1, 2 and 3
> Plan the specific elements of the programme
> Follow the service user's journey through the programme from entry to exit
> Establish the cost of programme delivery: pay and non-pay
> Write up the programme proposal
> Consider a small pilot or phased implementation plan
> Commence programme delivery
> Plan and complete an evaluation of the programme
> Write up a manual of the final programme
> Share the programme and the lessons learned with others

- The extent of unemployment among those with early psychosis
- The right to work
- The economic benefits of return to employment

The importance of work to society

Many Western cultures are very work-orientated. One only has to consider what is inferred by the question 'what do you do?' to gain an indication of how work is regarded by society. Typically, paid work (employment) is held in high regard and unpaid work (parenting, studying, volunteering) is regarded as valuable by most, whereas those not working (unemployed) and particularly those not willing to work can be resented by other members of society (Fryers, 2006). Paid employment is the common means of achieving adequate economic resources which are essential for people to fully participate in society. Without employment the risk of social exclusion and poverty is dramatically increased and according to Evans and Repper (2000), 'poverty, unemployment, social exclusion and mental health are intricately linked' (p. 15). High unemployment among those affected by mental health problems perpetuates the negative attitudes unaffected people already hold. The lack of people in the workforce with disclosed mental health problems provides 'evidence' that a mental health problem renders a person unable to work (Evans & Repper, 2000). Some employers acknowledge they are less likely to give a job to someone who discloses they have mental health problems (National Economic and Social Forum, 2007). This lack of access to one of the most common routes for a positive community presence and valued status in society further compounds the challenges people with mental illness face.

However, just as unemployment can 'disable' a person, return to employment 'enables' someone through providing an income for fuller participation in society, extending the social network and providing a positive answer to the question often asked 'what you do you?'; in essence, employment facilitates the person to become socially included rather than excluded.

The importance of work to people recovering from psychosis

It is only in the last decade that a substantive body of research on the opinions of people with serious mental illness regarding work has emerged. Unsurprisingly, the findings mirror the opinions of the general population; people with serious mental illness, including young people recovering from their first experience of psychosis, consider work to be of great importance (Bassett et al., 2001; Kennedy-Jones et al., 2005; Marwaha & Johnson, 2005; Provencher et al., 2002) and critical to recovery (Dunn et al., 2008). The importance of occupation, of being engaged in and having aspirations for meaningful occupational roles and goals, was also highlighted by the young people with psychosis who participated in the evaluation of the TIME programme of early intervention (Fisher & Savin-Baden, 2001). Just like members of the community without mental illness, people with mental illness want to work (South Essex Service Research Group, Secker & Gelling, 2006) and view not working as leading to a lack of money, inactivity and not perceiving themselves as being 'well' (Reid et al., 1993, cited in Evans & Repper, 2000).

The benefits of employment and the perils of worklessness

The benefits of employment and perils of worklessness do not stop at a social level but also impact on our physical and mental health. According to Shortt (1996), unemployment is in itself pathogenic with many ill effects on health. Specifically, the review determined that the most common disorders associated with unemployment are emotional and cardiopulmonary diseases, particularly among the younger people, the economically marginal and middle-age men (Shortt, 1996). However, although the corollary might be assumed – that work is beneficial to health – the evidence had not been reviewed and published until recently. Waddell and Burton (2006) reviewed the evidence for the UK Health, Work and Well-Being Strategy and conclude that 'there is a strong evidence base showing that work is generally good for physical and mental health and well-being. Work can be therapeutic and can reverse the adverse health effects of unemployment' (p. ix). With regard to severe mental illness in particular, the review does not conclude that employment causes improved health; however, on the balance of indirect evidence it regards work as beneficial for overall well-being and, importantly, that work is not harmful to the mental health of those with severe mental illness. A recent randomised control trial of supported employment also provides evidence that employment does not lead to increased hospital use and, as the authors suggest, should reassure clinicians who are concerned that those returning to work would relapse due to the stresses of employment (Burns et al., 2007).

Rates of unemployment among those with early psychosis

Low rates of employment are not just confined to people with enduring schizophrenia but are also seen among people experiencing their first episode of psychosis. The review on employment and schizophrenia by Marwaha and Johnson (2004) included first-episode psychosis studies published up to 2002. Employment rates at baseline ranged from 25 to 65%. Rates of employment at follow-up ranged from 16% at 3 years to 49% at 2-year follow-up. Unfortunately, there is evidence of rising unemployment over time in some studies. A 5-year follow-up with first-time patients seeking help for psychosis in three catchment areas in Stockholm, Sweden, reported work functioning at four time periods: Week 1, Year 1, 3 and 5. Results show that at Week 1 4% of the 71 participants were on disability allowance, at Year 1 this had risen to 11%, at Year 3 to 39% and at Year 5 to 52% (Svedberg et al., 2001).

The right to work

Article 23 of the Universal Declaration of Human Rights (1948) contains four parts:

(1) Everyone has the right to work, to free choice of employment, to just and favourable conditions of work and to protection against unemployment.

(2) Everyone, without any discrimination, has the right to equal pay for equal work.

(3) Everyone who works has the right to just and favourable remuneration ensuring for himself and his family an existence worthy of human dignity, and supplemented, if necessary, by other means of social protection.

(4) Everyone has the right to form and to join trade unions for the protection of his interests.

Members of the United Nations are expected to attempt to achieve this common standard for all the people of its state and where applicable other territories for which it is responsible. The International Covenant on Economic, Social and Cultural Rights (1966) also supports an individual's right to work in the context of individual freedoms and economic, social and cultural development. Article 6 states:

(1) The State Parties to the present Covenant recognize the right to work, which includes the right of everyone to the opportunity to gain his living by work, which he freely chooses or accepts, and will take appropriate steps to safeguard this right.
(2) The steps to be taken by a State party to the present Covenant to achieve the full realization of this right shall include technical and vocational guidance and training programmes, policies and techniques to achieve steady economic, social and cultural development and full and productive employment under conditions safeguarding fundamental political and economic freedoms to the individual.

The African Charter on Human and Peoples' Rights (1981) also recognises the right to work, emphasising conditions and pay. Article 15 states:

Every individual shall have the right to work under equitable and satisfactory conditions, and shall receive equal pay for equal work.

However, the low rates of employment among many marginalised groups and lack of effort to tackle discrimination of people with conditions misunderstood by society like schizophrenia indicates that these rights are not a reality for 'everyone' as these declarations state, and there is relatively little effort being made to redress the situation. It will require vocational rehabilitation practitioners to highlight these injustices and ensure that people with mental health problems receive the services required for them to attain employment free from discrimination.

The economic benefits of improving employment outcomes

There is increasing awareness of the large contribution that lost productivity makes to the overall cost of schizophrenia; in one study 42% of the total cost of the illness was determined to be the result of unemployment (Behan et al., 2008). Without employment a person cannot generate a financial income for themselves or for society. It is this loss of tax revenue that leads to this high cost associated with unemployment. There are also the secondary costs of providing social welfare payments to those not in paid work. The high potential economic gain of successful employment interventions can increase their attractiveness to service providers and funding bodies and therefore should be included in a vocational programme proposal.

Vocational programmes for early psychosis with an emerging evidence base

Supported employment, in particular the Individual Placement and Support model (IPS), has developed a considerable evidence base in the last 10 years (Drake & Bond, 2008). Eleven randomised control trials in four different continents – North America, Europe, Asia and Australia – have been conducted (Bond et al., 2008). The superior outcomes for recipients of supported employment point to a more widespread introduction of the model, yet investment is scarce outside the US. According to the World Health Organization, a combination of early intervention and supported employment is a natural progression in improving the employment outcomes of people with psychotic conditions (Marshall, 2005).

Rinaldi et al. (2004) evaluated the effectiveness of IPS in an early intervention service. With a half-time vocational specialist integrated into the Early Treatment and Home-based Outreach Service, there were significant increases in the proportion of clients engaged in work or educational activity over the first 6 months of the intervention, and in a subsample over a second 6-month period. Although 55% of the 40 participants were unemployed/unoccupied at baseline, only 7% had not achieved purposeful occupation at 6 months. Killackey et al. (2008) subjected IPS in an early intervention setting to a more rigorous test, through a randomised control trial of 41 people with first-episode psychosis conducted in the early intervention service in Melbourne, Australia. Twenty people received 6 months of IPS plus treatment as usual and 21 people received treatment as usual alone through random assignment. The IPS group had significantly better outcomes on level of employment, hours worked per week, jobs acquired and longevity of employment. The IPS group also significantly reduced their reliance on welfare benefits.

However, employment may not always be the most appropriate occupational avenue for someone recovering from early psychosis; completing education may be of greater interest. Like returning to employment, returning to education poses challenges; a person who wishes to return to education may need assistance in order to successfully achieve their goal. Not unlike supported employment, supported education is a model to assist people gain access to and be successful in post-secondary education (Unger, 1990). However, as a result of the scarcity of research there is little standardisation of approach (Carlson et al., 2003, cited in Corrigan et al., 2007) but ten features of supported education programmes have emerged through the evolution of the intervention to guide programme development and implementation (Waghorn et al., 2004). Supported education is discussed in detail in Chapter 15. Returning to education has been shown to have a number of benefits to those with long-term mental health problems including decreased perception of being stigmatised, increase in self-esteem, social functioning, independence, cognitive abilities, assertiveness and confidence. Furthermore, in-patient and day-patient hospitalisation rates of people who return to college can decrease, thereby offsetting the cost associated with providing a supported education programme (Isenwater et al., 2002).

Recently, there has been some blending of supported employment and supported education where the integrated vocational specialist delivering supported employment includes assisting those who wish to return to education to achieve their goal and then support them to maintain their student role (Nuechterlein et al., 2008). A randomised control trial of IPS ($n = 46$), which was extended to include supported education, was conducted with people with recent-onset schizophrenia (Nuechterlein et al., 2008). Published results indicate that of those randomised to IPS who successfully returned to work or education, 36% returned to education alone, 31% returned to employment alone and 33% returned to a combination of education and employment.

Nuechterlein et al. (2008) also provide us with an indication of (a) the extent and type of support people recently diagnosed with schizophrenia want and (b) their levels of comfort with regard to contact with employers and disclosure.

Extent of support: Only a minority (26%) of participants received 'behind the scenes' assistance, whereas 74% required the IPS specialist to play an active role in setting up job interviews, contacting schools to help complete the admission process, transporting participants to interview and in some instances sitting in on interviews. This relatively high level of support is important to take into consideration when planning caseload size and manpower of a supported employment/supported education programme.

Disclosure and contact with employers: Options were available for participants regarding the IPS specialist making contact with schools or employers, ranging from no permission to make contact to contact and attendance with the person at their place of work or school. Also permissible extent of disclosure was agreed, ranging from no disclosure of information to full disclosure of a psychiatric condition if the IPS specialist deemed it necessary. Participants' level of comfort with contact and disclosure varied widely and also changed over time. Specifically with regard to contact, initially 28% prohibited all contact, 31% permitted discussion of job or school performance with employers or teachers and 41% permitted discussion and observation of school or work performance. However by 18 months, 74% consented to the IPS specialist having contact with schools or employers. Regarding disclosure, 54% prohibited any disclosure of disability or psychiatric condition, 20% approved disclosure of a disability but not a psychiatric condition and 26% approved the disclosure of their psychiatric condition. During the trial, the need to disclose did not occur frequently (26%) and did not hinder the IPS specialist work, so it was not possible to determine whether participants would have allowed disclosure if necessary or did their position on the matter change over time.

Real world examples of vocational programmes in early intervention for psychosis services

The views of young people affected by psychosis are critical when developing a vocational rehabilitation programme for young people with psychosis. The findings of the study of Bassett et al. (2001) with a group of young people recently diagnosed with psychosis highlighted the barriers young people perceive they face when returning to work. The perceived difficulties emerging from their responses were:

- Loss, including loss of self-esteem, confidence, goals and abilities
- Stigma attached to mental illness that would affect employers' perception of them
- Treatment issues such as a lack of a collaborative approach from clinicians; symptom management, particularly in the workplace
- Life goals which are disrupted and now require revisiting
- The need for support from services to prepare them for return to work following a period of being unoccupied

People with psychosis have also expressed their views with regard to 'enablers' of successful return to work:

- The presence of a significant other, someone who provides consistent support and a sense of hope and belief that getting a job is feasible (Kennedy-Jones et al., 2005)
- The possibility of finding a job that matches a person's preferences, strengths and goals (Smith, 2000)

Vocational programmes are more likely to be successful if they address the barriers and include the enablers in as far as possible. However, they may also need to include elements not reported directly by young people affected by psychosis but have been established by research as associated with employment outcome, for example addressing cognitive functioning difficulties.

How to maximise the likelihood of success

A review of the factors associated with positive employment outcomes is beyond the scope of this chapter; however, a number of issues particularly important for early psychosis are important to mention.

A vocational programme cannot address pre-morbid adjustment difficulties or the absence of previous employment experience; however, there are opportunities to maximise the likelihood of a positive employment outcome by:

- Keeping delays to effective treatment as short as possible (Norman et al., 2007)
- Building a person's levels of motivation and self-efficacy (Grove & Membrey, 2005)
- Providing cognitive remediation (McGurk & Wykes, 2008)
- adopting supported employment approaches (Killackey et al., 2008)
- adopting an optimistic attitude towards the potential of the person achieving their vocational goals

Real World Example I

The Canadian early intervention service PEPP developed the COST (Cognitively Oriented Skills Training) group due to the significant cognitive deficits many people with psychosis present with and the importance of cognitive functioning for community functioning including employment (Malla et al., 2003). The COST group is designed to address deficits in functioningthat relate to academic performance through teaching cognitive and behavioural compensatory strategies for specific cognitive domains. The specific objectives of the COST group are:

- Increase the use and effectiveness of study strategies
- Decrease the frequency of cognitive complaints
- Improve attention and concentration
- Increase the use of memory and learning strategies
- Improve academic performance

These objectives are covered in ten 2-hour sessions, one per week. There is usually a 4:1 participant-to-therapist ratio (Malla et al., 2003)

Real World Example II

The Occupational Therapy (OT) service of Dublin and East Treatment and Early Care Team (DETECT) is provided on a one-to-one basis to those unoccupied when they present to the service. Following the completion of a standardised assessment process (see Box 9.2) the occupational therapist assists the person in setting and achieving personally meaningful goals within the areas of productivity, social and leisure skills, self-care and community living skills.

The intervention is primarily individual psychosocial sessions, during which goal setting and strategic planning are key components, working towards

---

Box 9.2   Standardised assessment process.

DETECT Occupational Therapy Assessment Protocol

Occupational Circumstances Assessment Interview and Rating Scale (OCAIRS)
Occupational Self-Assessment (OSA)
Kohlman Evaluation of Living Skills (KELS) [adapted for use with first-episode clients)
Life Skills Profile (LSP) [completed by telephone with next of kin]

---

linking in with various community agencies that will be of assistance. The principal area of need and therefore intervention is productivity, including pre-vocational skill building, job seeking, gaining and maintaining employment or voluntary work, and assistance re-entering education or training. Daily structure and leisure skills, including social and physical activities, are addressed with most clients, while other areas of intervention include stress management and relaxation techniques, community living skills and self-care issues. Over a 12-month period, of the 20 people who were successfully discharged from the OT service, 9 commenced a training course, 6 entered paid employment, 3 continued with their role as full-time parents and 2 were transferred to other mental health services (O'Leary & Turner, 2008).

Real World Example III

The Graduated Recovery Intervention Program (GRIP) for first-episode psychosis is a comprehensive, flexible cognitive-behavioural therapy programme that aims to enhance illness management and facilitate functional recovery following a first episode of psychosis. GRIP is provided to an individual, on a weekly basis, for up to 36 sessions and is composed of four phases:

(1) Engagement and wellness management
(2) Substance use
(3) Persistent symptoms
(4) Functional recovery

In addition to phase-specific content, the GRIP places an emphasis in all sessions on personal goal pursuit to foster optimism and self-esteem and on the enlistment of external social support to maximise therapeutic gains and engagement. The first 12 sessions of GRIP covering psychoeducation, goal setting, illness management and relapse prevention are relatively standardised. After 12 sessions have been completed, progress is evaluated and the client and the therapist collaboratively determine whether additional treatment is necessary. The remaining sessions are flexible and individually tailored to the needs of the client. Therapists are encouraged to follow the prescribed order of treatment phases; however, pressing client concerns are always prioritised, regardless of phase. In an open trial of ten participants in the GRIP, 67% were engaged with the programme for more than 12 sessions. Of these engagers the collective rate of goal attainment was 68% of their personal goals rated as 'very close to being achieved' or 'achieved' at post-test review, whereas none of the treatment non-completers' goals received those same ratings. Examples of goals that completers achieved during participation in GRIP include returning to school, making new friends, taking medication daily and learning more about mental illness (Waldheter et al., 2008).

Measuring success of vocational intervention for early psychosis

Increasingly, evidence of the efficacy of interventions provided by health services is necessary for continued support from sources of funding. Without evidence the continued delivery of interventions can be called into question, as was the conclusion of the recent review of the efficacy of life skills programmes (Tung-punkom & Nicol, 2008). Vocational interventions are increasingly evaluated based on hard employment outcomes such as rate of successful return to employment, average number of hours employed, salary earned, tax contribution and welfare savings. However, as mentioned earlier, defining employment is problematic. In some studies, employment includes students and those maintaining a home on a full-time basis; however, not all studies do the same. These difficulties were raised by Marwaha and Johnson (2004) and subsequently by Killackey et al. (2006). No two studies use the same method of categorisation in the first-episode studies reviewed by Marwaha and Johnson (2004).

A possible solution is a three-level categorical variable – employed, non-labour force work, unemployed – and may be useful for comparing employment/unemployment rates among people with psychosis to census data. This method allows the labour force of the sample to be calculated; that is, the labour force of a country (or other geographic entity) consists of everyone of working age (typically above a certain age (around 14–16) and below retirement age) who are participating workers, i.e. people actively employed or looking for work. The fraction of the labour force who is seeking work but cannot find it determines the unemployment rate. Turner et al. (2009) used this approach to categorise 162 people with first-episode psychosis. Of the whole sample, 46% were employed within the last month, 21% were engaged in non-labour force activities, such as study or parenting and therefore not seeking employment, and 33% were unemployed. When you subtract the non-labour force group

from the overall sample and express the number of the labour force not engaged in employment activity as a rate, the percentage unemployed is 42%,
nine times the local unemployment rate at the same time.

Cost-effectiveness is central to the evaluation of interventions and is often
regarded as the most important part of the evaluation by funding bodies. Due
to the high proportion of the cost of mental illnesses being attributable to
unemployment and under-employment, vocational rehabilitation programmes
that improve hard employment outcomes are keenly sought. Cost-effectiveness
takes into account not only the benefits in terms of hard employment outcomes
but also the cost of delivering the service. In order to conduct an accurate
cost-effectiveness study programme, providers must gather detailed 'accounts'
of both outcome and expenditure, which will require planning from the outset
of commencing the programme. The recent combined approach of supported
employment and supported education works in the best interest of the person
who requires vocational assistance; indeed, educational attainment is associated
with positive employment outcome (Waghorn et al., 2004). However, it poses
an interesting methodological cost-effectiveness study question as there are no
short-term social welfare savings or tax revenue generated from those who have
received input from the vocational specialist to attain and maintain education
or training; however, there may be long-term gains after the study has finished.
It may therefore appear that the intervention is not cost-effective when in fact
it is. Possibly in short-term cost-effectiveness studies of this combined model
excluding the positive outcome of attaining education and deducting the cost of
the hours the vocational specialist spends delivering supported education from
the cost of service delivery would lead to a more accurate results in terms of
cost-effectiveness.

Randomised control trials are regarded as the gold standard of establishing
the efficacy of interventions. To date, with the exception of supported employment, there have been relatively few trials of adequate power to evaluate
vocational rehabilitation programmes for people with early psychosis. Future
research that evaluates the effectiveness of one vocational programme compared to an equal amount of another approach will shed further light on the
best methodologies for assisting people recovering from early psychosis return
to work or education. Results of such evaluations will provide evidence that
service planners and funders will find difficult to ignore.

Conclusions

Return to work or education is unsurprisingly a priority for young people recovering from early psychosis. Traditionally such goals would often have gone
unattained; however, some positive developments now challenge the classic
negative occupational outcome. Developing and evaluating vocational recovery

programmes is an arduous task, but enabling people attain their occupational aspirations is critical to their recovery and future well-being. Without such programmes the high unemployment rates and associated problems currently reported among people with schizophrenia will continue. Early intervention services and evidence-based rehabilitation programmes are two key contributing factors to improving outcomes; however, their availability is scarce, particularly together in one service, although this is changing. Although IPS has evidence to support its introduction with young people with psychosis, it may be premature to stop developing and evaluating other innovative vocational rehabilitation approaches to accomplish the ambition of assisting all those recovering from psychosis to find a meaningful life.

References

African Charter on Human and Peoples' Rights (1981). Available at: http://en. wikipedia.org/wiki/African_Charter_on_Human_and_Peoples%27_Rights (accessed 28 April 2009).

Barnes, T.R., Hutton, S.B., Chapman, M.J., Mutsatsa, S., Puri, B.K., & Joyce, E.M. (2000). West London first-episode study of schizophrenia: clinical correlates of duration of untreated psychosis. *British Journal of Psychiatry*, 177, 207–211.

Bassett, J., Lloyd, C., & Bassett, H. (2001) Work issues for young people with psychosis: barriers to employment. *British Journal of Occupational Therapy*, 64, 66–72.

Behan, C., Kennelly, B., & O'Callaghan, E. (2008). The economic cost of schizophrenia in Ireland: a cost of illness study. *Irish Journal of Psychological Medicine*, 25, 80–87.

Birchwood, M., Todd, P., & Jackson, C. (1998). Early intervention in psychosis: the critical period hypothesis. *British Journal of Psychiatry*, 172, 53–59.

Boardman, J. (2003). Work, employment and psychiatric disability. *Advances in Psychiatric Treatment*, 9, 327–334.

Bond, G.R., Drake, R.E., & Becker, D.R. (2008). An update on randomized control trials of evidence based supported employment. *Psychiatric Rehabilitation Journal*, 31, 280–290.

Browne, S., Clarke, M., Gervin, M., Waddington, J.L., Larkin, C., & O'Callaghan, E. (2000). Determinants of quality of life at first presentation with schizophrenia. *British Journal of Psychiatry*, 176, 173–176.

Burns, T., Catty, J., Becker, T., Drake, R.E., Fioritti, A., Knapp, M., Lauber, C., Rössler, W., Tomov, T., van Busschbach, J., White, S., Wiersma, D., & EQOLISE Group (2007). The effectiveness of supported employment for people with severe mental illness: a randomised controlled trial. *Lancet*, 29, 1146–1152.

Chong, S.A., Mythily, S., & Verma, S. (2005). Reducing the duration of untreated psychosis and changing help-seeking behaviour in Singapore. *Social Psychiatry and Psychiatric Epidemiology*, 40, 619–621.

Clarke, M., & O'Callaghan, E. (2003). Is earlier better? At the beginning of schizophrenia: timing and opportunities for early intervention. *Psychiatric Clinics of North America*, 26, 65–83.

Clarke, M., Whitty, P., Browne, S., McTigue, O., Kinsella, A., Waddington, J.L., Larkin, C., & O'Callaghan, E. (2006). Suicidality in first episode psychosis. *Schizophrenia Research*, 86, 221–225.

Cook, J.A., Leff, H.S., Blyler, C.R., Gold, P.B., Goldberg, R.W., Mueser, K.T., Toprac M.G., McFarlane, W.R., Shafer, M.S., Blankertz, L.E., Dudek, K., Razzano, L.A., Grey, D.D., & Burke-Miller, J. (2005). Results of a multisite randomized trial of supported employment interventions for individuals with severe mental illness. *Archives of General Psychiatry*, 62, 505–512.

Corrigan, P.W., Mueser, K.T., Bond, G.R., Drake, R.E., & Solomon, P. (2007). *Principles and Practice of Psychiatric Rehabilitation: An Empirical Approach*. New York: Guildford Press.

Craig, T.K., Garety, P., Power, P., Rahaman, N., Colbert, S., Fornells-Ambrojo, M., & Dunn, G. (2004). The Lambeth Early Onset (LEO) Team: randomised controlled trial of the effectiveness of specialised care for early psychosis. *British Medical Journal*, 329, 1067.

Crowther, R., Marshall, M., Bond, G., & Huxley, P. (2001). Vocational rehabilitation for people with severe mental illness. *Cochrane Database Systematic Reviews*, Issue 2, Art. No. CD003080.

Drake, R.E., & Bond, G.R. (2008). Supported employment: 1998–2008. *Psychiatric Rehabilitation Journal*, 31, 274–276.

Dunn, E.C., Wewiorski, N.J., & Rogers E.S. (2008). The meaning and importance of employment to people in recovery from serious mental illness: results of a qualitative study. *Psychiatric Rehabilitation Journal*, 32, 59–62.

Evans, J., & Repper, J. (2000). Employment, social inclusion and mental health. *Journal of Psychiatric Mental and Health Nursing*, 7, 15–24.

Fisher, A., & Savin-Baden, M. (2001). An evaluation of the benefits to young people with psychosis, and their families, of an early intervention programme. *British Journal of Occupational Therapy*, 64, 58–65.

Friis, S., Vaglum, P., Haahr, U., Johannessen, J.O., Larsen, T.K., Melle, I., Opjordsmoen, S., Rund, B.R., Simonsen, E., & McGlashan, T.H. (2005) Effect of an early detection programme on duration of untreated psychosis: part of the Scandinavian TIPS study. *British Journal of Psychiatry*, 48, s29–s32.

Fryers, T. (2006) Work, identity and health. *Clinical Practice and Epidemiology in Mental Health*, 2, 12. Available at: www.cpementalhealth.com/content/2/1/12 (accessed 2 February 2009).

Grove, B., & Membrey, H. (2005). Sheep and goats: new thinking on employability. In: Grove, B., Secker, J., & Seebohm, P.R. (eds) *New Thinking about Mental Health and Employment*. Oxon: Radcliffe Publishing, UK, pp. 3–10.

International Covenant on Economic, Social and Cultural Rights (1966). Available at: http://en.wikipedia.org/wiki/International_Covenant_on_Economic_Social_and_Cultural_Rights (accessed 28 April 2009)

Isenwater, W., Lanham, W., & Thornhill, H. (2002). The College Link Program: evaluation of a supported education initiative in Great Britain. *Psychiatric Rehabilitation Journal*, 26, 43–50.

Kennedy-Jones, M., Cooper, J., & Fossey, E. (2005). Developing a worker role: stories of four people with mental illness. *Australian Journal of Occupational Therapy*, 52, 116–126.

Killackey, E.J., Jackson, H.J., Gleeson, J., Hickie, I.B., & McGorry, P.D. (2006). Exciting career opportunity beckons! Early intervention and vocational rehabilitation in first-episode psychosis: employing cautious optimism. *Australian and New Zealand Journal of Psychiatry*, 40, 951–962.

Killackey, E., Jackson, H.J., & McGorry, P.D. (2008). Vocational intervention in first-episode psychosis: individual placement and support v. treatment as usual. *British Journal of Psychiatry*, 193, 114–120.

Lindgren, I., Hogstedt, M.F., & Cullberg, J. (2006). Outpatient vs. comprehensive first-episode psychosis services, a 5-year follow-up of Soteria Nacka. *Nordic Journal of Psychiatry*, 60, 405–409.

Malla, A., Norman, R., McLean, T., Scholten, D., & Townsend, L. (2003). A Canadian programme for early intervention in non-affective psychotic disorders. *Australian and New Zealand Journal of Psychiatry*, 37, 407–413.

Marshall, M. (2005). How effective are different types of day care services for people with severe mental disorders? Copenhagen, WHO Regional Office for Europe (Health Evidence Network report. Available at: http://www.euro.who.int/Document/E87317.pdf (accessed 30 September 2008).

Marshall, M., Lewis, S., Lockwood, A., Drake, R., Jones, P., & Croudace, T. (2005). Association between duration of untreated psychosis and outcome in cohorts of first-episode patients: a systematic review. *Archives of General Psychiatry*, 62, 975–983.

Marwaha, S., & Johnson, S. (2004). Schizophrenia and employment – a review. *Social Psychiatry and Psychiatric Epidemiology*, 39, 337–349.

Marwaha, S., & Johnson, S. (2005) Views and experiences of employment among people with psychosis: a qualitative descriptive study. *The International Journal of Social Psychiatry*, 51, 302–316.

McGorry, P.D., Edwards, J., Mihalopoulos, C., Harrigan, S.M., & Jackson, H.J. (1996). EPPIC: an evolving system of early detection and optimal management. *Schizophrenia Bulletin*, 22, 305–326.

McGorry, P.D, Killackey, E., & Yung, A. (2007). Early intervention in psychotic disorders: detection and treatment of the first episode and the critical early stages. *Medical Journal of Australia*, 187, S8–S10.

McGurk, S.R., & Wykes, T. (2008) Cognitive remediation and vocational rehabilitation. *Psychiatric Rehabilitation Journal*, 31, 350–359.

Melle, I., Larsen, T.K., Haahr, U., Friis, S., Johannessen, J.O., Opjordsmoen, S., Simonsen, E., Rund, B.R., Vaglum, P., & McGlashan, T. (2004). Reducing the duration of untreated first-episode psychosis: effects on clinical presentation. *Archives of General Psychiatry*, 61, 143–150.

National Economic and Social Forum (2007). *Mental Health in the Workplace: Research Findings*. Dublin: National Economic and Social Forum.

Norman, R.M., Mallal, A.K., Manchanda, R., Windell, D., Harricharan, R., Takhar, J., & Northcott, S. (2007). Does treatment delay predict occupational functioning in first-episode psychosis? *Schizophrenia Research*, 91, 259–262.

Nuechterlein, K.H., Subotnik, K.L., Turner, L.R., Ventura, J., Becker, D.R., & Drake, R.E. (2008). Individual placement and support for individuals with recent-onset schizophrenia: integrating supported education and supported employment. *Psychiatric Rehabilitation Journal*, 31, 340–349.

O'Leary, T., & Turner, N. (2008). The role of occupational therapy in an Irish early intervention service for psychosis. *Irish Journal of Occupational Therapy*, 36, 22–28.

Perkins, R., & Rinaldi, M. (2002). Unemployment rates among patients with long term mental health problems. *Psychiatric Bulletin*, 26, 295–298.

Petersen, L., Nordentoft, M., Jeppesen, P., Ohlenschaeger, J., Thorup, A., Christensen, T.Ø., Krarup, G., Dahlstrøm, J., Haastrup, B., & Jørgensen, P. (2005). Improving 1-year outcome in first-episode psychosis: OPUS trial. *British Journal of Psychiatry*, *48*, s98–s103.

Provencher, H.L., Gregg, R., Mead, S., & Mueser, K.T. (2002). The role of work in the recovery of persons with psychiatric disabilities. *Psychiatric Rehabilitation Journal*, *26*, 132–144.

Rinaldi, M., McNeil, K., Firn, M., Koletsi, M., Perkins, R., & Singh, S.P. (2004). What are the benefits of evidence-based supported employment for patients with first-episode psychosis? *Psychiatric Bulletin*, *28*, 281–284.

Shortt, S.E. (1996). Is unemployment pathogenic? A review of current concepts with lessons for policy planners. *International Journal of Health Services: Planning, Administration and Evaluation*, *26*, 569–589.

Smith, M.K. (2000). Recovery from severe psychiatric disability: findings of a qualitative study. *Psychiatric Rehabilitation Journal*, *24*, 149–158.

South Essex Service Research Group, Secker, J., & Gelling, L. (2006) Still dreaming: service users' employment, education and training goals. *Journal of Mental Health*, *15*, 103–111.

Svedberg, B., Mesterton, A., & Cullberg, J. (2001). First-episode non-affective psychosis in a total urban population: a 5-year follow-up. *Social Psychiatry and Psychiatric Epidemiology*, *36*, 332–337.

The International First Episode Vocational Recovery Group (2008). *Meaningful Lives: International Consensus Statement*. Available at: http://www.iris-initiative.org.uk/promote-recovery-and-ordinary-lives/recovery-and-ordinary-lives/international-consensus-statement.html (accessed 3 March 2009).

Tungpunkom, P., & Nicol, M. (2008). Life skills programmes for chronic mental illnesses. *Cochrane Database of Systematic Reviews*, Issue 2, Art. No. CD000381.

Turner, N., Browne, S., Clarke, M., Gervin, M., Larkin, C., Waddington, J.L., & O'Callaghan, E. (2009). Employment status amongst those with psychosis at first presentation. *Social Psychiatry and Psychiatric Epidemiology*, *44*, 863–869.

Turner, N., Jackson, D., Renwick, L., Sutton, M., Foley, S., McWilliams, S., Kinsella, A., & O'Callaghan, E. (2007). What influences purpose in life in first-episode psychosis? *British Journal of Occupational Therapy*, *70*, 401–406.

Universal Declaration of Human Rights (1948). Available at: http://en.wikipedia.org/wiki/Universal_Declaration_of_Human_Rights (accessed 28 April 2009).

Unger, K. (1990). Supported postsecondary education for people with mental illness. *American Rehabilitation*, *16*, 19–31.

Waddell, G., & Burton, K. (2006). *Is Work Good for Your Health and Wellbeing?* Norwich: TSO (The Stationery Office).

Waghorn, G., Still, M., Chant, D., & Whiteford, H. (2004). Specialised supported education for Australians with psychotic disorders. *Australian Journal of Social Issues*, *39*, 443–458.

Waldheter, E.J., Penn, D.L., Perkins, D.O., Mueser, K.T., Whaley Owens, L., & Cook, E. (2008). The Graduated Recovery Intervention Program for first episode psychosis: treatment development and preliminary data. *Community Mental Health Journal*, *44*, 443–455.

Whitty, P., Clarke, M., McTigue, O., Browne, S., Kamali, M., Kinsella, A., Larkin, C., & O'Callaghan, E. (2008). Predictors of outcome over the first four years of illness in first episode schizophrenia. *Psychological Medicine*, *38*, 1141–1146.

Chapter 10

WORK-RELATED SOCIAL SKILLS AND JOB RETENTION

Hector W.H. Tsang and Sally M.Y. Li

Chapter overview

Work is generally beneficial to health and quality of life, and it has been found that unemployment has adverse effects on people. To assist people find work, the most evidence-based approach used is that of supported employment (SE), particularly the Individual Placement and Support (IPS) approach. It has been found that while the success rate of IPS is impressive based on research results, there is still a substantial proportion of clients who fail in the process of securing or maintaining employment. The most-often reported problems are interpersonal difficulty and inability to cope with the job demands. This chapter discusses work-related social skills training and how it may be used to enhance vocational outcomes. A study is reported which found more successful job finding amongst participants who attended a programme which combined social skills with vocational assistance.

Work-related social skills and job retention

Work has long been regarded as a potential contributor and a tool for the treatment of mental illness (Ekdawi et al., 1994). It is an uppermost part of life and has many advantages for people, which include supplying a source of income, providing a source of social identity and status, social contacts and support, and offering a sense of personal achievement (Rinaldi et al., 2004). Unemployment on the contrary has demonstrated adverse effects on health caused by poverty, poor housing and a rejection by society (Brenner, 1987; Smith, 1987). While work serves a range of important functions in a person's life, not every person, however, can enjoy the benefits of work, particularly those suffering from schizophrenia and other major psychoses. There are various reasons that cause unemployment of people with severe mental illness (SMI), which include poor pre-morbid occupational performance, lack of working experiences, poor social skills or social functioning level, and deficits in cognitive functioning (Tsang et al., 2000a).

Social skills and social competence

Studies show that social behaviour at work is a critical factor for successful employment of people with mental illness (Argyle, 1992; Carpenter & Strauss, 1991; Lysaker et al., 1995; Solinski et al., 1992). Unfortunately, the employment problem can result when people with schizophrenia lack the appropriate social competence and social skills necessary in the workplace (Rudrud et al., 1984; Tsang, 2003; Tsang & Pearson, 2000).

Social skills are a group of behaviours which people need in order to interact and communicate effectively with others. Social rules and relations are created, communicated and developed in verbal and non-verbal ways. They involve receiving skill, which is to correctly identify desired outcomes and emotion; processing skill, which is to generate alternatives and their consequences; and sending skill, which includes verbal and non-verbal components so that our thoughts and ideas can be expressed and exchanged with others. Social competence refers to being able to possess and use these skills to integrate thinking, feeling and behaviour to produce the desired outcomes on other people in social situations. These include perception and interpretation of social cues, anticipation of obstacles to personally desired behaviour, anticipation of consequences of behaviour for self and others, generation of effective solutions to interpersonal problems, translation of social decisions into effective social behaviours and the expression of a positive sense of self-efficacy. Generally speaking, social competence is 'being able to get on with other people'. It involves the ability to establish, maintain and develop friendly relationships with other people, be cooperative and helpful, and be able to communicate clearly and to persuade others to do things in working contexts and in our own personal lives (Argyle & Kendon, 1976).

The importance of social skills in work situations is well documented (Argyle, 1992; Fontana, 1990; Tsang 2003; Tsang & Pearson, 2000). Social skills and social competence play a critical role in the process of job search and retention. It is an essential element for a successful employment which may improve the quality of life of people with SMI. Unfortunately, people with SMI usually fail in competitive employment due to a lack of the social competence and social skills necessary in the workplace (Lignugaris-Kraft et al., 1988; Rudrud et al., 1984; Turner, 1977). It is obvious that any form of employment involves interpersonal relationships and contacts with supervisors, fellow workers and customers. There are two phases of the employment process: acquiring a job and maintaining a job. Each phase has different interpersonal demands and thus needs different social skills. The job searching stage needs the skills of locating available jobs, interview skills and skills of acclimating to an unfamiliar environment. In contrast, the job maintenance phase requires that one performs the task requirement of the job and gets along with others for a long period of time. Social skill deficits presented among people with schizophrenia include making eye contact, carrying on a conversation and expressing appropriate affect (Mueser et al., 1991). Such social skills deficits contribute to the unemployment of people with SMI.

Work-related social skills

Although social behaviours are essential for acquiring and maintaining gainful employment, there has not been a comprehensive understanding on 'work-related social skills' (WSS). Different authors tend to interpret the term in different ways. Argyle (1992), for instance, listed six categories of skills required of an employee: reasoned arguments, ingratiation, exchange of benefits, assertiveness, appeal to a higher authority and forming a coalition. Fontana (1990) proposed five basic social skills that are essential for a worker to win a good first impression from others in the workplace: remembering names, holding conversations, making self-disclosures, giving praise and encouragement and showing agreement. Foy et al. (1979) listed another five components of skills necessary at work. These were compliance, requesting changes, speech duration, percentage of eye contact and overall assertiveness. However, a unified and consistent interpretation among the theorists and practitioners is lacking. It is certain from the authors cited above that WSS involves several variables including basic social skills, skills in interaction with seniors, fellow workers and subordinate, and skills in handling special work situations. A more systemic schema for WSS can be found in a paper by Salzberg et al. (1988), who used the term 'social-vocational competence', consisting of task-related and personal-social competence, instead of WSS. Although this model appears to be fairly systematic, it is by no means complete and directly applicable to the rehabilitation of those with SMI. Apart from the components included in the above discussion, it is strongly felt that job-securing social skills and skills in handling job situations specific to a particular job surely also are domains of concern for WSS.

As mentioned above, an important employment problem of people with SMI is a lack of social competence and social skills necessary in the workplace. The problems include not knowing how to deal with criticisms from the supervisor, how to serve customers and how to deal with stigmatising attitude from co-workers. People with SMI usually experience social skills deficits, which may affect their valued life and lead to a failure of employment. Thus, WSS training is developed for people with SMI, which emphasises on improving their abilities in handling interpersonal challenges with co-workers and supervisors. The strategy involves helping clients achieve vocational goals in various stages of job seeking and actual employment. Tsang (2001) has developed a work-related social skill training (WSST) for people with psychiatric problems. WSST is conceptualised within a three-tier framework comprising basic skills, core skills and the results subsequent to the possession of these skills. This approach implies that the three tiers have a hierarchical relationship, with the first tier being more basic and the other two tiers being more advanced.

The first tier is composed of basic social skills and basic social survival skills. Basic social skills, which include skills related to the receiving, processing and sending of information (Liberman et al., 1986), and assertiveness focus on interpersonal communication. Basic social survival skills consist of such skills as grooming, politeness and personal appearance, which are necessary for social competence. The second tier is composed of two clusters of core skills component: skills in handling general work-related situations and skills in handling specific work-related situations. The first cluster includes those skills required for coping with any job irrespective of its special nature. General work-related skills can be divided into job-securing social skills and job-retaining skills. The second cluster comprises skills vital for coping with situations specific to a particular kind of job. Finally, the third tier encompasses the results to which the basic and core skills point: in other words, the benefits that a person can obtain if he or she possesses these skills. The benefits embrace getting a job, settling down in a job, maintaining a job and deriving a sense of achievement and satisfaction from the job.

Job tenure of people with severe mental illness

There are various approaches of vocational rehabilitation that have been used to improve the employment outcomes of people with SMI. The most evidence-based approach is SE, particularly the IPS approach (Drake & Becker, 1996). The principles of the IPS model are integration of vocational and clinical services; rapid job search; matching jobs to customers' preferences, skills and experiences; and time-unlimited job supports (Drake & Becker, 1996). Although the success rate of the IPS clients is shown to be impressive on the basis of available research results, there were still nearly half of the participants who failed in the process of securing competitive employment. It has been reported that persons with SMI had difficulty in maintaining jobs rather than finding jobs (Cook, 1992; MacDonald-Wilson et al., 1991; Xie et al., 1997). There are many factors contributing to the difficulties, which include a lack of work experience and poor social skills (Anthony & Jansen, 1984), inadequate supports (Cook, 1992) and stressful environment (Bond, 1994). Furthermore, studies showed that many people with SMI experience unsatisfactory job terminations, which is defined as client quitting the job without having other job plans or simply being fired (Cook, 1992; Fabian & Wiedefeld, 1989; MacDonald-Wilson et al., 1991).

Several studies revealed the reasons of job terminations among the participants of the SE programme. The most frequently reported problems were interpersonal difficulty and inability to cope with the job demand (Becker et al., 1998; Wong et al., 2001). Becker et al. (1998) found that there are multiple problems associated with unsatisfied job terminations, which included interpersonal functioning (58%), mental illness (52%), dissatisfaction with the job (52%), quality of work (36%), medical illnesses (30%), dependability (22%) and substance abuse (15%). This is in line with the available evidence in the literature (Cook & Razzano, 2000; Tsang et al., 2000a), which has shown that social competence is one of the most significant predictors of employment outcome among individuals with mental illness.

Social competence and job tenure

Social competence plays a significant role in vocational functioning and employment outcomes among people with SMI. In a review of previous cross-sectional and longitudinal studies, it is concluded that the relationship between social and vocational functioning is well established (Bond et al., 1998). However, the theoretical account linking the relationship between social and vocational functioning on people with SMI is extremely limited. There are at least two reasons for this knowledge gap. Firstly, there is the neglect of the fact that accommodation in the workplace is a social process (Gates, 2000). Most of the traditional vocational rehabilitation approaches view accommodation as technical changes to job tasks, job routines or the physical environment. The interpersonal aspect of the accommodation is largely neglected. Examples include how to interact with supervisor and co-workers, and how to deal with customers. Secondly, there is little attempt to conceptualise social skills needed for job acquisition and retention among people with mental illness.

Predictors of employment outcomes of individuals with psychiatric disabilities have continued to be studied since the 1960s. It sheds light on the relationship between social competence and employment outcomes. A review of the literature from 1985 to 1997 (Tsang et al., 2000a) found that social skills received consistent support as a significant predictor of employment outcome. It was found that social skills show a very high correlation with overall employability. In a 14-year longitudinal follow-up study conducted in Germany (Vetter & Koller, 1996), social functioning was found to be one of the three strongest predictors of occupational development in a group of 214 patients. Studies recently conducted in Hong Kong reported similar results. A survey carried out among medical and rehabilitation professionals ($N = 118$) at a mental hospital showed that it was generally perceived that social competence in general and in the workplace were strong predictors of vocational outcome (Tsang et al., 2000b). In another study by Tsang and Pearson (1996), a survey was conducted among 44 rehabilitation professionals and 54 clients with schizophrenia in halfway houses and sheltered workshops. The majority of the respondents thought that being socially competent was an important factor for successful employment of people suffering from schizophrenia.

A study (Tsang et al., 2000c) showed that the employed clients scored significantly higher than the unemployed in social and general behaviours of the Workshop Behavior Checklist. There was no significant difference in scores of vocational behaviours. As to the scores of the Vocational Social Skills Scale, the scores of the employed and unemployed clients differed only in basic social survival skills. There was no difference in scores on perceived social competence, basic social skills and situation-specific social skills. This suggests that for people with SMI, it is easier to obtain a job if they have better basic social survival skills, which are the most fundamental skills necessary for seeking and keeping a job. To conclude, poorer vocational outcomes are associated with poorer social skills in people with SMI.

In discussing the role of social skills in the workplace, Bond et al. (1998) commented that the job acquisition process includes locating available jobs, successfully interviewing for a job and acclimating to an unfamiliar setting, whereas job retention requires skills in getting along with others for an extended period of time. From the above discussion, it is clear that the failure of people with SMI in getting and maintaining a job may be due to problems related to their social functioning. Therefore, it is important to help clients to master social skills in the vocational context.

Work-related social skills training

Although social skills training is a well-established treatment modality for people with schizophrenia which helps improve their social competence (Penn & Mueser, 1996), its potential benefit to augment the vocational outcome of SE has not been explored. A recent and more systematic attempt to adopt the skills training approach to help persons with serious mental illness maintain their jobs is the 'workplace fundamentals' developed by Wallace et al. (1999). The reason for developing this module is simply that SE showed no advantage over traditional vocational rehabilitation services in helping workers retain their jobs. The skill areas covered in the module include identifying how work changes participants' lives, using problem solving to manage symptoms and medications at the workplace, learning how to interface with supervisors and peers to improve job task performance, and using problem solving to recruit social support on and off the job.

Another training module to improve their social skills necessary for getting and keeping a job is based on a conceptual framework put forward and validated by Tsang and Pearson (1996) and the UCLA basic principles of social skills training (Liberman et al., 1989). This is a ten-session work-related social skills training module (Tsang & Pearson, 2001) which is a structured and manualised programme to teach clients job interview skills, basic conversation and social survival skills for effective communication with supervisor, co-workers and customers. WSST consists of ten-group sessions, with each session lasting 1.5–2 hours. Clients first receive training on verbal and non-verbal communication, accurate social perception, assertiveness, grooming and personal appearance, greetings and other basic conversation skills. Afterwards, they proceed to the core work-related skills in special situations in the workplace such as handling conflicts and requesting sick leave, and also problem-solving skills. Each session of the WSST follows the standard components of the social skills training, including warm-up activities, instructions, demonstrations, role-plays, feedbacks and homework assignments (Liberman et al., 1989; Wallace et al., 1980).

Enhancing vocational outcomes of SE

IPS is an evidence-based rehabilitation service that includes job development and placement, ongoing employment supports, coordination of vocational services with multidisciplinary treatment teams, indefinite services and the opportunity for choice of jobs by participants. Success rates average over 50% employment during the course of a 6-month period of IPS. However, IPS is less than optimal in clients maintaining their jobs, with 50% of those employed experiencing job terminations at the 6-month follow-up. Over a longer follow-up period, considerably fewer than half of the participants in IPS are working during any single month (Bond et al., 1997).

To improve vocational outcomes from IPS, various enhanced versions (Gold et al., 2006; McGurk et al., 2005; Mueser et al., 2005; Wallace, 2004) were developed by augmenting IPS with additional psychosocial interventions. We developed an Integrated Supported Employment (ISE) programme, which combines IPS with social skills training, an evidence-based treatment that has been shown to improve social communication, social problem solving and social functioning in persons with schizophrenia and other disabling mental disorders (Kopelowicz et al., 2006; Kurtz & Mueser, 2008). The choice of social skills training was inspired by the fact that interpersonal difficulties have been found to be the most frequently reported job problem leading to unwanted job terminations (Becker et al., 1998). In addition, social competence has been found to be a significant predictor of gainful employment. The service protocol of ISE follows the steps of the IPS prototype programme (Becker & Drake, 1993), which include (1) referral, (2) building a relationship, (3) vocational assessment, (4) individual employment plan, (5) obtaining employment and (6) follow-along support. Social skills training is part of the ISE approach during vocational assessment. Assessment on social skills necessary for seeking and maintaining a job is incorporated into the ISE. In employment plan formulation, an emphasis is on the role social skills play in the individual employment plan. Before obtaining employment, the WSST module (Tsang & Pearson, 2001) will be used. Ongoing includes an emphasis on providing assistance to the clients how to develop and maintain good and cooperative working relationship with their fellow workers, supervisors and customers.

To test its effectiveness, a 15-month randomised controlled trial (RCT) of ISE was conducted in Hong Kong (Tsang et al., 2009). Between 2003 and 2005, 163 participants from community mental health programmes which offered a range of rehabilitation services were recruited. The recruitment was based on the following selection criteria: (1) suffering from SMI (operationally defined as schizophrenia, schizoaffective disorder, bipolar disorder, recurrent major depression or borderline personality disorder); (2) being unemployed; (3) willing and cognitively competent to give informed consent; (4) lacking obvious cognitive, learning and neurological impairments as determined by mental status exam; (5) completed primary education; and (6) expressing a desire to work. The subjects were randomly assigned to ISE, IPS and TVR (traditional vocational rehabilitation) using SPSS. There were no statistically significant differences among the three groups in gender, educational level, diagnosis and employment history. The outcome measures of the study included the vocational aspects (i.e. employment rate, job tenure, salary and number of job terminations) and psychosocial aspects. Employment Outcome Checklist (EOC), the 21-item Chinese Job Stress Coping Scale (CJSC) and the Chinese Job Termination Checklist (CJTC) were used as the outcome measures. The programme lasted for 15 months for the ISE and IPS groups from programme admission to completion of the follow-up support. The TVR group received traditional vocational service for 15 months, which mirrored the other two groups. Assessment using the instruments listed above was conducted by an independent, trained and blind assessor with an occupational therapy background at programme admission (baseline), completion of the 3-month programme, and follow-up at 7, 11 and 15 months.

We obtained an employment rate of 78.8% among the ISE participants at the 15th month since joining the service, which was significantly higher than that among the IPS participants (53.6%). As social competence is a significant predictor of employment outcome (Tsang et al., 2000a, c; Vetter & Koller, 1996), it makes sense that more ISE participants with special training in job-seeking skills gained competitive employment than did IPS participants. Factors contributing to more successful job finding among the ISE participants were probably due to the improved job interview skills acquired during the WSST sessions. Their performance was appraised by the employment specialist (ES) after each job interview so that the participants learned from their own mistakes. In addition, the ES helped the participants make improvements for their future performance. Furthermore, the impressive results that we obtained in this study may be partially because employers would put more weight on social skills of the job applicants in Hong Kong and Chinese culture when they make hiring decisions. A cross-cultural study on employers' concerns on hiring people for entry-level jobs has provided support to this as the study has shown that employers in China pay more attention to interpersonal skills and solidarity of applicants when compared with employers in the USA (Tsang et al., 2007). To conclude, our findings demonstrated that the WSST module combined with IPS was able to boost up the employment rate of people with SMI.

Other than the employment rate, the RCT found that the job tenure of ISE participants averaged 24 weeks, which was 12 weeks longer than that of the IPS participants towards the end of the follow-up period at 15th month after the commencement of the programme. As discussed by Tsang (2003), social skills play a critical role in the process of job search and retention among people with SMI. In the study of Lehman et al. (2002), there was no between-group difference in the length of employment between IPS participants and ISE participants. Lehman hypothesised that impaired interpersonal skills played a significant role in job retention problems. The major difference between ISE and IPS was that the social functioning of the participants was enhanced in the ISE programme by a social skills training module and the efforts targeted at skills generalisation throughout the entire follow-along process. Job-retaining social skills including maintaining a good working relationship with the supervisor and co-workers were imparted to the participants (Tsang, 2003). These social skills equipped them with ways to cope with the interpersonal conflicts in the workplace that might cause participants to leave the jobs. Follow-along support of the ISE programme focused on improving and maintaining the relationship with their supervisor or co-workers and emphasis was given to the generalisation of the social skills they learned. Whenever ISE participants had problems with their supervisor or co-workers, the employment specialist reminded them of the social skills learned in the work-related social skills training programme. The employment specialist set the behavioural goal together with the participants. The behavioural goal was specific and related to the workplace of the participants such as building up relationships with supervisors and co-workers when they started a new job, or maintaining and improving social relationships in workplace if they had conflicts or interpersonal difficulties. The employment specialist discussed with the participants appropriate behaviours in dealing with the social problems using a social problem-solving approach, performed behavioural rehearsal and provided practical assistance to the participants so that they could bridge the gap in generalising the skills to their workplace. Both the behavioural goal and the specific behaviours were recorded to remind them of the goals and behaviours. The specialist met them regularly and reviewed their performance. If the participants could handle the interpersonal difficulties successfully, reinforcement was given as encouragement. At the same time, the employment specialist discussed with the participants about upgrading the behavioural goals. On the other hand, if they could not handle the problems well, the specialist provided further assistance and practised with them again until they were able to deal with the work situations. Although our IPS participants also received similar service (e.g. practical advice from the employment specialist and discussion of the problem using a problem-solving approach) during the follow-up period, it was not conducted using the skills training approach to target for more behavioural improvement as in the ISE intervention protocol. The results of this study supported that improving the social functioning of people with mental illness via a brief skills training programme before they enter the competitive job market and skill generalisation strategies helping them cope with their interpersonal conflicts after they have secured a job could lengthen their job duration.

In addition, the reasons of job terminations of both IPS participants and ISE participants were investigated. As to the reasons of job terminations, 25.0% of the IPS participants were related to interpersonal problems. The result was consistent with Becker et al.'s study (Becker et al., 1998) that a lot of job problems pertained to interpersonal difficulty. However, only 7.7% of the ISE participants terminated their jobs because of social problems in workplace. Although a significant difference in terms of interpersonal reasons between IPS and ISE was not achieved at this stage, the obvious trend was that ISE participants had less interpersonal difficulties in the workplace than IPS participants.

Case illustration of ISE

Mr. Chan was a 44-year-old gentleman who suffered from paranoid schizophrenia since 2000. He had been unemployed for over 2 years before he was referred to the ISE team by a non-governmental organisation. He did not know what kinds of jobs would be suitable for him.

In the first meeting, the employment specialist introduced the purposes of the ISE service and the employment specialist's role in the ISE service protocol. The employment specialist explained how ISE could help Mr. Chan in job hunting and dealing with his difficulties in the workplace.

The employment specialist initiated assessment to evaluate how well Mr. Chan could work in a competitive job in the community. The employment specialist assessed Mr. Chan's educational background, work history, work skills, strengths and weaknesses, and preference. In addition, the employment specialist assessed his social competence in getting and holding a job. According to his work history, he had worked in different roles such as laboratory assistant and salesperson. He started investing in properties and stock in 1995. However, he lost all his money from 1997 to 1999. Then he worked as a financial planner. But he quitted the job later due to the stress he experienced resulting from the demanding nature of his field. During the period of onset, he felt being persecuted and the telephone line was hooked by triad society members. Finally, he was admitted to a psychiatric hospital due to psychotic relapse and high anxiety level. The employment specialist also obtained information on Mr. Chan's likes, dislikes and job preferences. He expressed that he felt easily agitated and was therefore unable to cope with highly demanding jobs. He described himself as a hardworking person but did not like to communicate with others. He possessed basic computer skills and hoped to find a clerical job.

The employment specialist then formulated an individual employment plan for Mr. Chan. Firstly, WSST was provided to enhance his social skills. He expressed that he wanted to obtain a clerical job. The ultimate goal of the individual employment plan was to maintain employment and prolong job tenure.

Mr. Chan lacked the necessary social skills and social competence to get and keep a job (Cook & Razzano, 2000; Tsang, 2003; Tsang & Pearson, 2001). Before the job search, Mr. Chan participated in the manualised WSST (Tsang, 2001) to enhance his ability to seek and maintain a job. Mr. Chan was very attentive and cooperative throughout the WSST. However, he was usually passive and did not comment on or join in the discussion with other participants. In the job interview skills session, Mr. Chan was required to look for a job advertisement according to his preference and role-play a job interview exercise. Throughout the process, Mr. Chan gradually gained better understanding on the requirements of clerical work in the competitive job market. He finally found a job advertisement for an office assistant, which met all his job requirements. Through demonstration and modelling, Mr. Chan was equipped with appropriate job interview skills and work-related social skills necessary for securing the job. He then practised these skills with the employment specialist so that his social skills could be consolidated and generalised from the WSST sessions to his workplace. Appreciation and encouragement were given to him after the role-play exercises to establish the motivation for learning and applying the skills. After ten WSST sessions, Mr. Chan's social skills had significantly improved and he was ready for seeking a job.

The employment specialist regularly accompanied Mr. Chan to the Labor Department to search for job vacancies and encouraged him to apply for jobs in which he was interested. Generalisation of the skills learned in WSST was applied to the process of obtaining employment, following the steps set out in Figure 10.1. The employment specialist encouraged Mr. Chan to prepare himself before each job interview by reviewing the WSST content regarding job interview skills. Mr. Chan's preference was an office assistant position. The employment specialist discussed this with Mr. Chan and set a behavioural goal with him to perform well during the interview and obtain the job. Through several guided practices he became more familiar with the interview process. Eventually he found a job as an office assistant.

An important task for the employment specialist at this stage is to help the client generalise the social skills learned in WSST and improve his relationship with the supervisor and co-workers. This task constitutes one of the most

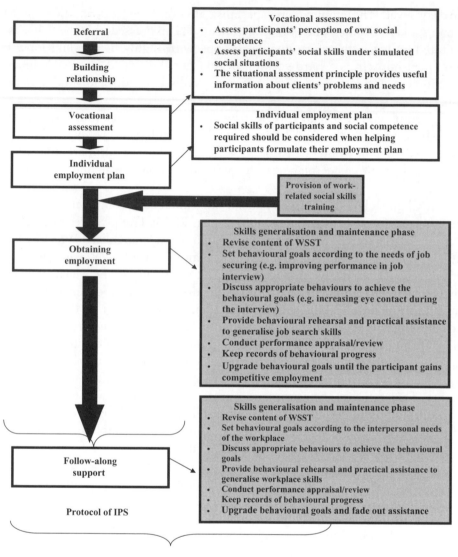

Figure 10.1 Protocol of Integrated Placement and Support (IPS) and Integrated Supported Employment (ISE).

important differences between ISE and IPS and accounts for ISE participants' longer job tenures (Tsang et al., 2009). The following sections illustrate how the employment specialist helped Mr. Chan cope with his interpersonal difficulties in the workplace.

Although Mr. Chan succeeded in getting the job, he was perplexed by the interpersonal difficulties he had with his supervisor. He complained that his supervisor was a picky and highly demanding person who piled stress on him. He was anxious during work and thus made a lot of mistakes. Mr. Chan avoided contact with his supervisor and sometimes responded to the job request in an impolite way.

To follow the protocol of the ISE, the employment specialist took prompt action and discussed with Mr. Chan on the reasons of the high demand of the supervisor. The employment specialist taught him how to report his problem to his supervisor using the social skills acquired in the WSST sessions. The employment specialist first reminded Mr. Chan of the WSST content regarding communicating with the supervisor. He was encouraged to utilise the social skills learned in his working place. The employment specialist set a behavioural goal together with Mr. Chan, which was to successfully seek advice from the supervisor. The employment specialist also discussed with Mr. Chan any appropriate behaviour that would facilitate him achieve the behavioural goal and help him perform the appropriate behaviours through role-play and performance appraisal. After completing guided exercises on several occasions, Mr. Chan was able to master the social skills to report problems to his supervisor and seek necessary help.

During the follow-up contact, Mr. Chan reported to the employment specialist that his supervisor understood his difficulties and allowed more time for him to finish the tasks. Finally, Mr. Chan was able to work in that company for more than 9 months and was satisfied with the job.

Conclusions

The effectiveness of the ISE programme in enhancing employment rates and job tenures among individuals with SMI has been well demonstrated by the 15-month RCT (Tsang et al., 2009). The major factors contributing to more successful job finding among the ISE participants are probably due to the improved social skills and social competence acquired during the WSST sessions and practised again during the follow-up. Clinicians should be encouraged to adopt such approaches for vocational rehabilitation among people with SMI.

References

Anthony, W.A., & Jansen, M.A. (1984). Predicting the vocational capacity of the chronically mentally ill: research and policy implications. *American Psychologist, 39*, 537–544.

Argyle, M. (1992). *The Social Psychology of Everyday Life.* New York: Routledge.

Argyle, M., & Kendon, A. (1976). The experimental analysis of social performance. *Advances in Experimental Social Psychology, 3*, 55–98.

Becker, D.R., & Drake, R.E. (1993). *A Working Life: The Individual Placement and Support (IPS) Program.* New Hampshire: Dartmouth Psychiatric Research Center.

Becker, D.R., Drake, R.E., Bond, G.R., Xie, H., Dain, B.J., & Harrison, K. (1998). Job terminations among persons with severe mental illness participating in supported employment. *Community Mental Health Journal, 34,* 71–82.

Bond, G.R. (1994). Applying psychiatric principles to employment: recent findings. In: Ancill, R.J., Holliday, S., & Higenbottam, J. (eds) *Schizophrenia: Exploring the Spectrum of Psychosis,* West Sussex, England: John Wiley & Sons, pp. 49–65.

Bond, G.R., Drake, R.E., & Becker, D.R. (1998). The role of social functioning in vocational rehabilitation. In: Mueser, K.T., & Tarrier, N. (eds). *Handbook of Social Functioning in Schizophrenia,* Boston: Allyn & Bacon, pp. 372–390.

Bond, G.R., Drake, R.E., Mueser, K.T., & Becker, D.R. (1997). An update on supported employment for people with severe mental illness. *Psychiatric Services, 48,* 335–346.

Brenner, M.A. (1987). Relation of economic and social well-being, 1950–1980. *Social Science Medicine, 25,* 183–196.

Carpenter, W.T., & Strauss, J.S. (1991). The prediction of outcome in schizophrenia. IV: Eleven-year follow-up of the Washington IPSS cohort. *The Journal of Nervous and Mental Disease, 179,* 517–524.

Cook, J.A. (1992). Job ending among youth and adults with severe mental illness. *The Journal of Mental Health Administration, 19,* 158–169.

Cook, J.A., & Razzano, L. (2000). Vocational rehabilitation for persons with schizophrenia: recent research and implications for practice. *Schizophrenia Bulletin, 39,* 42–53.

Drake, R.E., & Becker, D.R. (1996). The individual placement and support model of supported employment. *Psychiatric Services, 47,* 473—475.

Ekdawi, M.Y., Conning, A.M., & Campling, J. (1994). *Psychiatric Rehabilitation: A Practical Guide.* London: Chapman & Hall.

Fabian, E.S., & Wiedefeld, M.F. (1989). Supported employment for severely psychiatrically disabled person: a descriptive study. *Psychosocial Rehabilitation Journal, 2,* 53–60.

Fontana, D. (1990). *Social Skills at Work.* Exeter, UK: BPCC.

Foy, D.W., Massey, F.H., Duer, J.D., Ross, J.M., & Wooen, L.S. (1979). Social skills training to improve alcoholics' vocational interpersonal competence. *Journal of Counseling Psychology, 26,* 128–132.

Gates, L.B. (2000). Workplace accommodation as a social process. *Journal of Occupational Rehabilitation, 10,* 85–98.

Gold, P.B., Meisler, N., Santos, A.B., Carnemolla, M.A., Williams, O.H., & Keleher, J. (2006). Randomized trial of supported employment integrated with assertive community treatment for rural adults with severe mental illness. *Schizophrenia Bulletin, 32,* 378–395.

Kopelowicz, A., Liberman, R.P., & Zarate, R. (2006). Recent advance in social skills training for schizophrenia. *Schizophrenia Bulletin, 32,* S12–S23.

Kurtz, M.M., & Mueser, K.T. (2008). A meta-analysis of controlled research on social skills training for schizophrenia. *Journal of Consulting and Clinical Psychology, 76,* 491–504.

Lehman, A.F., Goldberg, R., Dixon, L.A., McNary, S., Postrado, L., Hackman, A., & McDonnell, K. (2002). Improving employment outcomes for persons with severe mental illnesses. *Archives of General Psychiatry, 59,* 165–172.

Liberman, R.P., DeRisi, W.J., & Mueser, H.K. (1989). *Social Skills Training for Psychiatric Patients.* New York: Pergamon Press.

Liberman, R.P., Mueser, K.T., Wallace, C.J., Jacobs, H.E., Eckman, T., & Massel, H.K. (1986). Training skills in the psychiatrically disabled: learning coping and competence. *Schizophrenia Bulletin, 12,* 631–647.

Lignugaris-Kraft, B., Salzberg, C.L., Rule, S., & Stowitschek, J.J. (1988). Social-vocational skills of workers with and without mental retardation in two community employment sites. *Mental Retardation, 26*, 297–305.

Lysaker, P.H., Bell, M.D., Zito, W.S., & Bioty, S.M. (1995). Deficits and predictors of improvement in schizophrenia. *The Journal of Nervous and Mental Disease, 183*, 688–691.

MacDonald-Wilson, K.L., Revell, W.G., Nguyen, N., & Peterson, M.E. (l991). Supported employment outcomes for people with psychiatric disability: a comparative analysis. *Journal of Vocational Rehabilitation, 1*, 30–44.

McGurk, S.R., Mueser, K.T., & Pascaris, A. (2005). Cognitive training and supported employment for persons with severe mental illness: one-year results from a randomized controlled trial. *Schizophrenia Bulletin, 31*, 898–909.

Mueser, K.T., Aalto, S., Becker, D.R., Ogden, J.S., Wolfe, R.S., Schiavo, D., Wallace, C.J., & Xie, H. (2005). The effectiveness of skills training for improving outcomes in supported employment. *Psychiatric Services, 56*, 1254–1260.

Mueser, K.T., Bellack, A.S., Douglas, M.S., & Morrison, R.L. (1991). Prevalence and stability of social skill deficits in schizophrenia. *Schizophrenia Research, 5*, 167–176.

Penn, D.L., & Mueser, K.T. (1996). Research update on the psychosocial treatment of schizophrenia. *American Journal of Psychiatry, 153*, 607–616.

Rinaldi, M., Mcneil, K., Firn, M., Koletsi, M., Perkins, R., & Singh, S.P. (2004). What are the benefits of evidence-based supported employment for patients with first-episode psychosis? *Psychiatric Bulletin, 28*, 281–284.

Rudrud, E.H., Ziarnik, J.P., Bernstein, G.S., & Ferrara, J.M. (1984). *Proactive Vocational Rehabilitation*. Baltimore, MD: Brookes.

Salzberg, S.S., Lignugaris/Kraft, B., & McCuller, G.L. (1988). Reasons for job loss: a review of employment termination studies of mentally retarded workers. *Research in Developmental Disabilities, 9*, 153–170.

Smith, R. (1987). *Unemployment and Health*. Oxford: Oxford University Press.

Solinski, S., Jackson, H.J., & Bell, R.C. (1992). Prediction of employability on schizophrenia patients. *Schizophrenia Research, 7*, 141–148.

Tsang, H., Lam, P., Ng, B., & Leung, O. (2000a). Predictors of employment outcome fo people with psychiatric disabilities: a review of the literature since mid 80s. *Journal of Rehabilitation, 66*, 19–31.

Tsang, H., Ng, B., IP, Y.C., & Mann, S. (2000c). Predictors of post-hospital employment status of persons with mental illness in Hong Kong: from perception of rehabilitation professionals to empirical evidence. *International Journal of Social Psychiatry, 46*, 306–312.

Tsang, H.W.H. (2001). Applying social skills training in the context of vocational rehabilitation for people with schizophrenia. *Journal of Nervous and Mental Disease, 189*, 90–98.

Tsang, H.W.H. (2003). Augmenting vocational outcomes of supported employment by social skills training. *Journal of Rehabilitation, 69*, 25–30.

Tsang, H.W.H, Angell, B., Corrigan, P.W., Kee, Y.T., Shi, K., Lam, C.S., Jin, S., & Fung, K.M.T. (2007). A cross-cultural study of employers' concerns about hiring people with psychotic disorder: implications for recovery. *Social Psychiatry and Psychiatric Epidemiology, 42*, 723–733.

Tsang, H.W.H., Chan, A., Wong, A., & Liberman, R.P. (2009). Vocational outcomes of an integrated supported employment program for individuals with persistent and severe mental illness. *Journal of Behavior Therapy and Experimental Psychiatry, 40*, 292–305.

Tsang, H.W.H., Lam, P., Dasari, B., Ng, B., & Chan, F. (2000b). Predictors of post-hospital employment status for psychiatric patients: perceptions of rehabilitation health professionals in Hong Kong. *Psychiatric Rehabilitation Journal, 24*, 169–173.

Tsang, H.W.H., & Pearson, V. (1996). A conceptual framework on work-related social skills for psychiatric rehabilitation. *Journal of Rehabilitaion, 69*, 25–30.

Tsang, H.W.H., & Pearson, V. (2000). Reliability and validity of a sample measure for assessing the social skills of people with schizophrenia necessary or seeking and securing a job. *Canadian Journal of Occupational Therapy, 67*, 250–259.

Tsang, H.W.H., & Pearson, V. (2001). Work-related social skills training for people with schizophrenia in Hong Kong. *Schizophrenia Bulletin, 27*, 139–148.

Turner, R.J. (1977). Jobs and schizophrenia. *Society Policy, 8*, 32–40.

Vetter, P., & Koller, O. (1996). Clinical and psychosocial variables in different diagnostic groups: their interrelationships and value as predictors of course and outcome during a 14-year follow-up. *Psychopathology, 29*, 159–168.

Wallace, C.J. (2004). Supplementing supported employment with workplace skills training. *Psychiatric Services, 55*, 513.

Wallace, C.J., Nelson, C.J., Liberman, R.P., Aitchison, L.D., Elder, J.P., & Ferris, U. (1980). A review and critique of social skills training with schizophrenic patients. *Schizophrenia Bulletin, 6*, 42–63.

Wallace, C.J., Tauber, R., & Wilde, J. (1999). Teaching fundamental workplace skills to persons with serious mental illness. *Psychiatric Services, 50*, 1147–1153.

Wong, K.K., Chiu, S.N., Chiu, L.P., & Tang, S.W. (2001). A supported competitive employment programme for individuals with chronic mental illness. *Hong Kong Journal of Psychiatry, 11*, 13–18.

Xie, H., Dain, B.J., Becker, D.R., & Drake, R.E. (1997). Job tenure among persons with severe mental illness. *Rehabilitation Counseling Bulletin, 40*, 230–239.

Chapter 11

WHEN SYMPTOMS AND TREATMENTS HINDER VOCATIONAL RECOVERY

Terry Krupa

Chapter overview

Any symptoms or impairments of a mental illness can interfere with employment, but some have consistently been associated with poorer vocational outcomes. These include negative symptoms, depression and cognitive impairments. Treatment factors that can interfere with vocational recovery include complications arising from medications. In addition, service providers may not prioritise employment in treatment planning because of assumptions about the relationship between working and mental illness. Current best practice offers a range of approaches and interventions to reduce the negative impact of symptoms and treatments on employment outcomes in mental illness including collaborative psychopharmacology, illness management, cognitive interventions, job matching, and the integration of vocational and clinical services. These approaches and interventions will have the greatest impact when they are integrated with comprehensive supported employment approaches.

Introduction

Ann has been working as a clerk in the health records department of a large general hospital for more than 20 years (Krupa, 2004). This is a job with responsibility, requiring her to perform a wide variety of tasks to ensure that the health records are in good order and can be accessed in a timely manner to facilitate patient care. The job requires her to stay abreast of technological changes related to health records management and large-scale reforms to the organization of the health care environment. By all accounts Ann has been an exemplary employee. She also happens to have a diagnosis of schizophrenia. Even though the illness is well treated by medications, Ann continues to experience symptoms of her illness, symptoms that can appear while she is working. For example, Ann occasionally experiences auditory hallucinations. Here Ann describes how these experiences can enter her work life, compromising the meaning she gives to social interactions at work:

> I treat [my co-workers] all the same. I'm very nice to them . . . I very rarely am ever angry or upset you know about what somebody might be saying, and that's one thing, even though they may be talking about me and I hear some-thing and I'm not quite sure if I actually heard it or not, so I don't act on it.

Ann's employment experiences bear similarities to many people who have a mental illness and desire employment. Despite the tremendous advancements in treatments for mental illness, many people will continue to experience some symptoms and impairments and these will impact them as they go about their day-to-day activities, including work. Ann's case highlights another important point: symptoms and impairments of mental illness are not always inconsistent with working, and many people develop the ability to manage these illness experiences in meaningful community employment.

In this chapter, symptoms and impairments of mental illness are defined according to the World Health Organization's International Classification of Functioning, Disability and Health (2001). Symptoms and impairments are located in the individual, and are significant deviations or loss of body functions. This chapter will examine:

- How symptoms of mental illness can hinder vocational recovery
- How treatment and services provided to people with mental illness can hinder their vocational recovery
- Approaches and interventions that can help to reduce the negative impact of these illness-related and clinical factors to promote vocational recovery

Background

Linking symptoms and impairments of mental illness to employment

The idea that mental illness impacts employment makes intuitive sense, but the nature of this relationship has proven very complex. Understanding the relationship between mental illness and employment recovery is complicated by the fact that vocational recovery actually comprises a broad range of outcomes and experiences. For example, vocational recovery might be defined by the extent to which employment is part-time or full-time, job tenure, the experience of satisfaction on the part of the employee, the level of payment provided for hours worked or even by the extent to which work holds the possibility for career advancement and socioeconomic prosperity. It may be that the impact of mental illness on employment is expressed through some outcomes, but not others. For example, Razzano et al. (2005) found that among research participants with serious mental illness, the specific diagnosis did not predict participation in employment, but it did predict intensity of working with those having a diagnosis of schizophrenia working fewer hours in a month.

Complicating our understanding further is the fact that illness-related factors may actually exert their influence on employment in ways that are not easily discernable. So, for example, in the study by Razzano et al. (2005), described above, the authors suggested that the lower numbers of hours worked by people with schizophrenia might be understood by the sedative effects of the anti-psychotic medications that they were likely prescribed. Yet, an alternate explanation might be that the apathy and avolition symptoms frequently experienced by people with schizophrenia, and to date poorly addressed by medication treatments, reduced the energy and commitment to work beyond a limited number of hours.

It would make sense that the severity of illness would be associated with poorer work outcomes, but again the relationship is unclear. Many mental illnesses such as affective disorders and schizophrenia are episodic in nature. In these cases, the experience of very acute symptoms and their negative impact on the ability to work may be time limited. Yet, where the course of the mental illness is of a long duration, then symptoms and impairments experienced below the level of acute illness may continue to impact work function. For example, Judd et al. (2008) studied the long-term course of depressive disorders and found that functioning at work was negatively associated with severity of depressive symptoms, and that even subthreshold levels of depressive symptoms appear to negatively impact functioning at work.

Diagnosis and employment outcomes

In Chapter 8 by Lloyd and Waghorn, the authors described how labour force participation is reduced for people with a wide range of mental disorders, with those experiencing illnesses with features of psychosis particularly disenfranchised from community work. Their findings are consistent with earlier research, indicating that people with schizophrenia, a mental illness characterised by features of psychosis, have poorer vocational outcomes compared to people with other psychiatric diagnoses (Wewiorski & Fabian, 2004). Yet, research to date has not consistently shown psychiatric diagnosis to be a predictor of who can or will work (Tsang et al., 2000). The evidence now available suggests that service systems and providers should not use diagnosis to determine who will benefit from employment supports to achieve vocational recovery.

How symptoms/impairments hinder employment

Any symptom associated with a mental illness can act as a barrier to employment (Waghorn & Lloyd, 2005). The nature of this interference will depend on the interaction between the individual's experiences of symptoms coupled with the actual work demands and context. So, for example, one young man might experience unmanageably high levels of anxiety when asked to give a public address in his job, while another living with post-traumatic stress disorder following a major vehicle accident may find himself unable to manage the highway driving demands of his job. It is possible for a person to work in a job where the demands rarely, or only minimally, collide with the symptoms or impairments of mental illness. Providing effective employment supports in mental health service delivery depends on service providers having a sound knowledge of mental illness, the ability to collaborate with an individual to identify important symptom patterns and the ability to analyse how specific work demands interact with symptoms to impact work performance and satisfaction.

There are specific symptoms and impairments that have been found to be generally predictive of poor employment outcomes and these are the focus of the remainder of this section. The constellation of symptoms known as negative symptoms of severe mental illnesses has been consistently linked to poorer employment outcomes (Razzano et al., 2005; Slade & Salkever, 2001; Tsang et al., 2000). People with negative symptoms demonstrate affective flattening, poverty of speech, avolition, impairments of attention and social withdrawal (Kay et al., 1987).Their experience of pleasure from activities is constrained, even when they attach meaning and value to those activities. This symptom constellation can present as a general disturbance in motivation and a reduction in personal drive, goal-directed behaviours and sustained investment towards a goal. In employment, this could translate into difficulties following through on an interest to work, a lack of attention to important work-related behaviours, discomfort in social relations at work and problems with sustaining the commitment to manage the inevitable challenges and demands that employment will present (Bond & Meyer, 1999; Cook & Razzano, 2000; Lysaker & Bell, 1995). While medications have demonstrated effectiveness in reducing positive symptoms of psychosis, such as hallucinations, they have been less successful in reducing negative symptoms.

Symptoms of depression have been associated with prolonged and severe work disability (Judd et al., 2008). Depression has been identified as a major health issue in the workplace, both because of the sheer numbers of employees and the economic costs to business (Dewa et al., 2004; Sederer & Clemens, 2003). Depression has also been linked to the work disability and lost work days experienced by people with a broad range of health issues such as diabetes (Egede, 2004), arthritis (Löwe et al., 2004) and low back pain (Pincus et al., 2002).

Depressive symptoms can rob an individual of the drive and the energy for work, and the ability to concentrate on work tasks. It can undermine personal confidence and self-esteem at work. A particular work productivity pattern that has been associated with depression is 'presenteeism' (Goetzel et al., 2004). Compared to absenteeism, which refers to the worker staying away from the job, presenteeism is defined as coming to work but performing below par. Current research is examining the nature of the work disability associated with depression. Studies have found that depression can negatively impact focus on work tasks (Wang et al., 2004) and create difficulties with mental-interpersonal tasks, time management and output tasks (Adler et al., 2006). Research by Lerner et al. (2004) has demonstrated that these disabilities translate into lost productivity in occupations that expect these particular proficiencies. Their research indicated, for example, that occupations with high demands for decision-making, communication and frequent interpersonal contacts with the public were particularly associated with loss of productivity in depression.

Cognitive impairments presenting in mental illness have also been associated with poorer employment outcomes (Tsang et al., 2000). Serious mental illnesses can lead to disturbances in several cognitive functions, such as personal insight, attention and concentration, working memory, processing speed, psychomotor speed and executive functioning that are fundamental to the task and social demands of contemporary work settings (McGurk & Meltzer, 2000; McGurk & Mueser, 2003, 2004). Jobs that are more complex, making frequent and significant demands on executive functioning, appear to be particularly demanding (McGurk & Mueser, 2003). Cognitive impairments may also impact employment by compromising social skills at work. Models of social skills have highlighted that good social functioning depends on an array of cognitive skills underlying the receiving, processing and sending of social messages (Tsang et al., 2000). Cognitive impairment can also complicate employment support services by limiting the rate of improvement that occurs in rehabilitation (Bell & Bryson, 2001).

How treatment hinders employment

Best practice in the treatment of many mental illnesses includes pharmacological treatments (Drake et al., 2001). These pharmacological treatments have had considerable success in reducing the symptoms associated with mental illness and preventing the relapse of acute exacerbations of illness – both important outcomes for facilitating positive employment outcomes. Leff and Warner (2006) highlight that by controlling the observable behaviours of symptoms, these medical treatments can reduce the public stigma and discrimination that can block access to important social roles such as employment.

Unfortunately, these pharmacological treatments can also have serious side effects that interfere with employment. For example, drugs used in the treatment of psychosis can cause drowsiness, sluggishness, shakiness and other disturbed movement patterns. They can also negatively impact spontaneity and motivation (Covell et al., 2007) that can have a direct impact on an individual's ability to perform work tasks or 'fit-in' socially on the job. As with medications for so many health conditions, those prescribed for mental illness may interfere with the ability to operate equipment. These unpleasant side effects of medications can compromise adherence to prescribed treatment regimens, which can impact the course of the mental disorders and threaten employment stability.

The new generation of atypical anti-psychotics has been found to have fewer side effects that interfere with function and they may reduce negative symptoms that have been particularly associated with poor employment outcomes (Lieberman et al., 2005). They may, however, present as barriers to employment in other ways. For example, one atypical medication, clozapine, has the potential to be lethal and requires regular blood testing. The need to attend frequent medical appointments could interfere with the individual's ability to maintain expected full-time work hours and to maintain privacy about having a health-related condition. Side effects such as weight gain associated with medications such as olanzapine (Lieberman et al., 2005) could compromise self-esteem and confidence and this may negatively impact work participation. These new generation medications can also be very expensive, and without a comprehensive health plan, paid employment may not be able to cover medication costs along with living expenses. This could compel individuals to apply for a government disability pension that provides both coverage for medications and a basic daily living allowance, but serves as a disincentive for participation in work (Stapleton et al., 2006).

There is evidence to suggest that employment is not prioritised as a desired outcome within mental health systems. Despite the advancements in the development of a range of effective employment supports, these are not routinely available or delivered within mental health service systems (Bertram & Howard, 2006; Blankertz & Robinson, 1996; Drake et al., 2003; Hanrahan et al., 2006).

Difficulties with advancing employment as a priority outcome in mental health service delivery arise from at least two traditionally held assumptions held within the mental health field. Firstly, there is the assumption that serious mental illnesses have a deteriorating course that is not consistent with the ability to work. This assumption continues to be present among service providers, even though there is now considerable evidence showing that the life course of mental illness is quite heterogeneous and that recovery of function in social roles, such as employment, is possible even after prolonged experiences of mental illness (Harding et al., 1987; Strauss, 2008).

Secondly, the field is influenced by well-established conceptual frameworks that assume that an underlying vulnerability to acute mental illness is exacerbated when the experience of stress overwhelms an individual's coping abilities (Anthony & Liberman, 1986). When mental health service providers view employment as a particularly demanding social role, with the potential to overwhelm the capacities of people with mental illness, work will not be prioritised and may in fact be discouraged (Krupa, 2004). Yet the nature of the relationship between stress and mental health is poorly understood, and certainly not in support of avoiding important and meaningful social roles.

Inconsistencies in the application of the stress-health association are frequent in the mental health field. For example, Marrone and Golowka (2005) argued that unemployment is at least as stressful as working, given the difficulties of poverty, lack of meaning and social isolation that it brings. Others have pointed out that the application of the 'vulnerability-stress' model of mental illness needs to consider important mediating factors such as the positive meaning given to work, the capacity of the individual to learn adaptive coping abilities and the potential for the social and task structure of work to be modified to enable performance (Anthony & Liberman, 1986). Indeed, contemporary perspectives on recovery from mental illness highlight that participation in work can be health promoting, and may have the capacity to reduce symptoms of mental illness (Krupa, 2004; Krupa et al., 2003).

In addition to these underlying assumptions, prioritising employment as an outcome in mental health service delivery can be impeded by a range of systemic and structural issues. Providers may lack knowledge and training in even basic evidence-based approaches to promoting employment. Job descriptions and rigidly enforced role distinctions among providers can limit access to employment support. Service protocols and resources may not be directed towards supporting employment. Nelson et al. (2001) direct three major criticisms to treatment services that can be applied to the area of employment. Firstly, they suggest that treatment services are routinely organised around professional expertise and not the needs and desires of the people served, including their desire for meaningful community-based work. Secondly, these treatment services rely on professional expertise to address problems, and are subsequently ill prepared to direct attention to the natural community resources and supports that might promote employment. Finally, these services may be housed in offices or institutions away from the communities where the people they serve live and work.

Approaches to reduce the negative impact of symptoms and treatments on vocational recovery

Collaborative pharmacological interventions

Decreasing the symptoms of mental illness through psychopharmacological treatments is considered a best practice in the routine delivery of mental health services (Drake et al., 2001, 2003; Mueser et al., 2003). Newer medications in the mental health arena have been developed with a view to reducing side effects and promoting function in the community. However, pharmacology has grown in complexity requiring the development of practice guidelines to ensure standards in practice. These guidelines outline the ranges for dosages, expected response times and identification of side effects (Mueser et al., 2003). Wang et al. (2004) have pointed out that pharmacological treatments do not consistently follow optimal recommended regimens and that this can be detrimental to employment.

A collaborative approach, actively involving people with mental illness in decision-making about medications, is considered an integral aspect of pharmacological treatment (Mueser et al., 2003). This collaborative approach may promote an individual's commitment to prescribed treatment regimens, be sensitive to funding issues for medications and promote the early identification of symptoms and side effects – all important to fulfilling work requirements.

Illness management approaches

Illness management includes a range of approaches designed to actively engage people in understanding and gaining control over the mental illness to reduce the risk of relapse and to enable successful participation in daily life roles and activities (Mueser et al., 2002). A hallmark of illness management strategies is the provision of education about mental illness and treatments. This education is frequently provided in a structured psychoeducational format, ensuring that people with mental illness are provided with standard knowledge about mental illness, the causes of mental illness and treatments with a view to encouraging their participation in decision-making and active problem solving (Mueser et al., 2002).

Psychoeducation has been offered to families of people with mental illness to provide them with the knowledge they need to enable them to promote quality and supportive family relationships. Research evidence has indicated that family psychoeducation can improve employment outcomes. It may be that psychoeducation better equips families to provide their member with mental illness with the support and living environment needed to manage employment (Dixon et al., 2000).

The evidence for the effectiveness of cognitive behavioural therapy (CBT) in the treatment of a range of mental illnesses is growing. CBT is a systematic approach to engaging people in recognising, changing and coping with underlying thought patterns that hinder their ability to participate in and enjoy daily life activities and roles. While the standardisation of CBT practices has developed, the actual application of CBT will depend on the nature of the symptoms experienced (Garety et al., 2000). Lysaker et al. (2005) developed a CBT intervention integrated within a programme of ongoing employment supports. Their intent was to provide a CBT intervention that would help people to develop new attitudes and beliefs about themselves as workers in order to overcome the hopelessness and emotional disengagement that interfere with the sustained commitment that employment requires. Research examining the effectiveness of this approach provides evidence for its positive impact on a range of employment outcomes and on hope, self-esteem and participant satisfaction (Davis et al., 2008; Lysaker et al., 2005).

Coping skills training focuses on developing the skills to manage symptoms and impairments as they emerge in the context of work. Krupa's (2004) study of employed workers with mental illness developed specific coping tasks that workers with mental illness engaged in to deal with symptoms on the job. For example, these tasks included vigilance for the early identification of thoughts, feelings and behaviours at work that might be signs of emerging mental illness, distinguishing between typical work experiences and those related to the illness, compensating for illness-related features on the job and interpreting work difficulties associated with illness as a part of the universal challenges of employment.

Wallace and Tauber (2004) describe a structured training programme for fundamental workplace skills that included problem solving and coping with problems related to symptoms, medications and other health issues on the job. The training was offered within a broader supported employment service, and thus was an adjunct to a full range of employment supports. The most notable finding of an initial study comparing this combined training-supported employment approach to supported employment alone was the greater job tenure and job satisfaction for the combined condition.

Cognitive interventions

To address the cognitive impairments that interfere with employment, several types of cognitive rehabilitation interventions have been developed. Cognitive remediation involves structured training, typically repetitive cognitive exercises, directed to improving specific weakened cognitive processes. Cognitive compensation, on the other hand, focuses on developing ways to minimise the impact of cognitive impairments in daily life. The use of a daily calendar to minimise problems with memory and written instructions to prompt the ordering of work tasks are examples of cognitive compensation. Increasingly, these specific interventions are being offered within full cognitive enhancement programmes, because of the complexity of these cognitive issues. Research on these interventions is encouraging with evidence emerging that cognitive function can be improved (Velligan et al., 2006).

Concerns have been raised about the extent to which cognitive interventions actually translate to improvements in participation in daily life roles. A promising response to this concern has been the creation of intervention programmes that integrate the performance of daily activities directly with cognitive interventions. For example, McGurk et al. (2005) describe a structured, combined cognitive remediation and compensation intervention called the 'Thinking Skills for Work Program', specifically designed for use within supported employment services. The intervention includes computer-based cognitive training, job search planning that carefully considers cognitive strengths, and ongoing consultation for cognitive issues as they emerge on the job. Their research on the effectiveness of the approach demonstrated improvements on a range of employment outcomes compared to the provision of employment supports alone.

Job matching

Individualised job matching can decrease the likelihood that the symptoms and impairments of a mental illness will hinder vocational recovery. This approach carefully considers the individual's unique interests, strengths and limitations in the selection and refinement of jobs (Kirsh et al., 2005). By attending to the preferences and interests of individuals, job matching can promote sustained motivation for work (Mueser et al., 2001). This may even serve to counteract some of the motivational problems experienced with negative symptoms.

Comprehensive job matching will include the analysis of the requirements of a job in relation to the individual's strengths and limitations in order to optimise the employment situation. This analysis can lead to informed decisions about the need for job modifications or specific work accommodations that can support employment when symptoms and impairments would otherwise hinder employment. In addition, this approach can include specific attention to the issue of how best to disclose to ensure accommodations while minimising stigma and discrimination in the workplace (Dalgin & Gilbride, 2003).

Integration of vocational and clinical services

Current best practice in employment support includes the integration of clinical and vocational services as a critical ingredient (Evans & Bond, 2008). This integration increases the capacity for clinical services to be responsive to treating symptoms and impairments of mental illness as they emerge at work and to refine these treatments to reduce the potential for side effects to interfere with employment. Integrated services can also ensure that co-occurring mental health issues, such as substance use, and coexisting health conditions, such as diabetes (both frequently experienced by people diagnosed with mental illness), are attended to in order to promote employment. Integration can also improve communication and problem solving in service delivery. For example, this close connection can encourage clinical service providers to more routinely consider employment planning in their work, and encourage providers of employment support to assertively extend their services to individuals who experience refractory symptoms and impairments.

The integration of clinical and vocational services is being supported within mental health systems, which are being reformed towards a recovery vision.

The concept of recovery suggests that mental health systems must create the conditions that are conducive to individuals with mental illness gaining the hope, healing, empowerment and connections to the larger social world that they require to live meaningful lives beyond the features that define mental illness (Jacobson & Greenley, 2001). The move to a recovery-oriented system also supports the development of formal peer-provider positions (Davidson et al., 2006). Certainly, many of the interventions and approaches described in this chapter could integrate peer-provider positions to capitalise on the lived experiences of people with mental illness, while assertively creating employment opportunities for people with mental illness.

Conclusions

Symptoms and impairments of mental illness and the problems inherent in treatment and service delivery represent illness and clinical factors that have the potential to hinder vocational recovery. The challenge of focusing on illness and clinical factors is that it encourages a 'deficit' view and compromises the ability to recognise the whole person, with strengths and potentials that can be optimised to promote employment. The example of Ann offered in the chapter's introduction is meant to remind that vocational recovery is possible even in the context of long-standing mental illness and marginalisation from the workforce. The approaches and interventions offered in this chapter provide an overview of several initiatives that have evidence supporting their success in promoting vocational recovery. These interventions will be most effective when they are integrated within a comprehensive service delivery package that includes a focus on promoting collaboration with individuals with mental illness and a full range of employment supports. We can expect that efforts to address these illness and clinical issues in vocational recovery will be advanced in the years to come.

References

Adler, D.A., McLaughlin, T.J., Rogers, W.H., Chang, H., Lapitsky, L., & Lerner, D. (2006). Job performance deficits due to depression. *American Journal of Psychiatry, 163*, 1569–1576.

Anthony, W.A., & Liberman, R.P. (1986). The practice of psychiatric rehabilitation: historical, conceptual and research base. *Schizophrenia Bulletin, 12*, 542–553.

Bell, M.D., & Bryson, G. (2001). Work rehabilitation in schizophrenia: does cognitive impairment limit improvement? *Schizophrenia Bulletin, 27*, 269–279.

Bertram, M., & Howard, L. (2006). Employment status and occupational care planning for people using mental health services. *Psychiatric Bulletin, 30*, 48–51.

Blankertz, R., & Robinson, S. (1996). Adding a vocational focus to mental health rehabilitation. *Psychiatric Services, 47*, 1216–1222.

Bond, G.R., & Meyer, P.S. (1999). The role of medications in the employment of people with schizophrenia. *Journal of Rehabilitation, 65,* 9–16.

Cook, J.A., & Razzano, L.A. (2000). Vocational rehabilitation for people with psychiatric disability. *American Rehabilitation, 20,* 2–12.

Covell, N.H., Weissman, E.M., Schell, B., McCorkle, B.H., Summerfelt, W.T., Weiden, P.J., & Essock, S. (2007). Distress with medication side effects among persons with severe mental illness. *Administration and Policy in Mental Health, 34,* 435–442.

Davidson, L., Chinman, M., Sells, D., & Rowe, M. (2006). Peer support among adults with serious mental illness: a report from the field. *Schizophrenia Bulletin, 32,* 443–450.

Davis, L.W., Ringer, J.M., Strasburger, A.M., & Lysaker, P.H. (2008). Participant evaluation of a CBT program for enhancing work function in schizophrenia. *Psychiatric Rehabilitation Journal, 32,* 55–58.

Dewa, C.S., Lesage, A., Goering, P., & Caveen, M. (2004). Nature and prevalence of mental illness in the workplace. *Healthcare Papers, 5,* 12–25.

Dalgin, R.S., & Gilbride, D. (2003). Perspectives of people with psychiatric disabilities on employment disclosure. *Psychiatric Rehabilitation Journal, 26,* 306–310.

Dixon, L., Adams, C., & Lucksted, A. (2000). Update on family psychoeducation for schizophrenia. *Schizophrenia Bulletin, 26,* 5–20.

Drake, R.E., Goldman, H.H., Leff, S., Lehamna, A.F., Dixon, L, Mueser, K.T., & Torrey, W.C. (2001). Implementing evidence-based practices in routine mental health service settings. *Psychiatric Services, 52,* 178–182.

Drake, R.E., Green, A.I., Mueser, K.T., & Goldman, H.H. (2003). The history of community mental health treatment and rehabilitation for persons with severe mental illness. *Community Mental Health Journal, 39,* 427–440.

Egede, L.E. (2004). Effects of depression on work loss and disability bed days in individuals with diabetes. *Diabetes Care, 27,* 1751–1754.

Evans, L.J., & Bond, G.R. (2008). Expert ratings on the critical ingredients of supported employment for people with severe mental illness. *Psychiatric Rehabilitation Journal, 31,* 318–331.

Garety, P.A., Fowler, D., & Kuipers, E. (2000). Cognitive-behavioral therapy for medication resistant symptoms. *Schizophrenia Bulletin, 26,* 73–86.

Goetzel, R.Z., Long, S.R., Ozminkowski, R.J., Hawkins, K., Wang, S., & Lynch, W. (2004). Health absence, disability and presenteeism cost estimates of certain physical and mental health conditions affecting U.S employers. *Journal of Occupational Environmental Medicine, 46,* 398–412.

Hanrahan, P., Heiser, W., Cooper, A.E., Oulvey, G., & Luchins, D.J. (2006). Limitations of system integration in providing employment services for persons with mental illness. *Administration and Policy in Mental Health and Mental Health Services Research, 33,* 244–252.

Harding, C.M., Brooks, G.W., Ashikaga, T., Strauss, J.S., & Breier, A. (1987). The Vermont longitudinal study of persons with severe mental illness. II: Long-term outcome of subjects who retrospectively met DSM-III criteria for schizophrenia. *American Journal of Psychiatry, 144,* 727–735.

Jacobson, N., & Greenley, D. (2001). What is recovery? A conceptual model and explication. *Psychiatric Services, 52,* 482–485.

Judd, L.L., Schettler, P.J., Solomon, D.A., Maser, J.D., Coryell, W., Endicott, J., & Akiskal, H.S. (2008). Psychosocial disability and work role function compared across the long-term course of bipolar I, bipolar II and unipolar major depressive disorders. *Journal of Affective Disorders, 108,* 49–58.

Kay, S.R., Fiszbein, A., & Opler, I. (1987). The Positive and Negative Syndrome Scale for schizophrenia. *Schizophrenia Bulletin*, *13*, 261–276.

Kirsh, B., Cockburn, L., & Gewurtz, R. (2005). Best practice in occupational therapy: program characteristics that influence vocational outcomes for people with serious mental illness. *Canadian Journal of Occupational Therapy*, *72*, 265–280.

Krupa, T. (2004). Employment, recovery and schizophrenia: integrating health and disorder at work. *Psychiatric Rehabilitation Journal*, *28*, 8–15.

Krupa, T., Zimolag, U., & Bond, G. (2003). How does work participation lead to clinical improvements in severe mental illness? In: 2003 *Making Gains Conference*, Toronto, Ontario. Available at: www.ontario.cmha.ca/making_gains.asp. (accessed 4 September 2008).

Leff, J., & Warner, R. (2006). *Social Inclusion of People with Mental Illness*. Cambridge, UK: Cambridge University Press.

Lerner, D., Adler, D.A., Chang, H., Berndt, E.R., Irish, J.T., Lapitsky, L., Hood, M.Y., Reed, J., & Rogers, W.H. (2004). The clinical and occupational correlates of work productivity loss among employed patients with depression. *Journal of Occupational and Environmental Medicine*, *46*, 1076–2752.

Lieberman, J.A., Stroup, T.S., McEvoy, J.P., Swartz, M.S., Rosenheck, R.A., Perkins, D.O., Keefe, R.S., Davis, S.M., Davis, C.E., Lebowitz, B.D., Severe, J., Hsiao, J.K.; Clinical Antipsychotic Trials of Intervention Effectiveness (CATIE) Investigators (2005). Effectiveness of antipsychotic drugs in patients with chronic schizophrenia. *The New England Journal of Medicine*, *353*, 1209–1223.

Löwe, B., Willand, L., Eich, W., Zipfel, S., Ho, A.D., Herzog, W., & Fiehn, C. (2004). Psychiatric comorbidity and work disability in patients with inflammatory rheumatic diseases. *Psychosomatic Medicine*, *66*, 395–402.

Lysaker, P., & Bell, M. (1995). Negative symptoms and vocational impairment in schizophrenia: repeated measurements of work performance over six months. *Acta Psychiatrica Scandinavica*, *91*, 205–208.

Lysaker, P.H., Bond, G., Davis, L.W., Bryson, G.J., & Bell, M.D. (2005). Enhanced cognitive-behavioral therapy for vocational rehabilitation in schizophrenia: effects on hope and work. *Journal of Rehabilitation Research and Development*, *42*, 673–682.

Marrone, J., & Golowka, E. (2005). If work makes people with mental illness sick, what do unemployment, poverty and social isolation cause? In: Davidson, L., Harding, C., & Spaniol, L. (eds) *Recovery from Severe Mental Illnesses: Research Evidence and Implications for Practice*, Vol. 1. Boston, MA: Center for Psychiatric Rehabilitation, pp. 451–463.

McGurk, S.R., & Meltzer, H.Y. (2000). The role of cognition in vocational functioning in schizophrenia. *Schizophrenia Research*, *45*, 175–184.

McGurk, S.R., & Mueser, K.T. (2003). Cognitive functioning and employment in severe mental illness. *The Journal of Nervous and Mental Disease*, *191*, 789–798.

McGurk, S.R., & Mueser, K.T. (2004). Cognitive functioning, symptoms and work in supported employment: a review and heuristic model. *Schizophrenia Research*, *68*, 1–27.

McGurk, S.R., Mueser, K.T., & Pascaris, A. (2005). Cognitive training and supported employment for persons with severe mental illness: one year results from a randomized controlled trial. *Schizophrenia Bulletin*, *31*, 898–909.

Mueser, K.T., Becker, D.R., & Wolfe, R. (2001). Supported employment, job preferences, job tenure and satisfaction. *Journal of Mental Health*, *10*, 411–417.

Mueser, K.T., Corrigan, P.W., Hilton, D.W., Tanzman, B., Schaub, A., Gingerich, S., Essock, S.M., Tarrier, N., Morey, B., Vogel-Scibilia, S., & Herz, M.I. (2002). Illness management and recovery: a review of the research. *Psychiatric Services*, *53*, 1272–1284.

Mueser, K.T., Torrey, W.C., Lynde, D., Singer, P., & Drake, R.E. (2003). Implementing evidence-based practices for people with severe mental illness. *Behaviour Modification*, 27, 387–411.

Nelson, G., Lord, J., & Ochocka, J. (2001). *Shifting the Paradigm in Community Mental Health*. Toronto: University of Toronto Press.

Pincus, T., Burton, K.A., Vogel, S., & Field, A.P. (2002). A systematic review of psychological factors as predictors of chronicity/disability in prospective cohorts of low back pain. *Spine*, 27, 109–120.

Razzano, L.A., Cook, J., Burke-Miller, J.K., Mueser, K.T., Pickett-Schenk, S.A., Grey, D.D., Goldberg, R.W., Blyler, C.R., Gold, P.B., Leff, H.S., Lehman, A.F., Shafer, M.S., Blankertz, L.E., McFarlane, W.R., Toprac, M.G., & Carey, M.A. (2005). Clinical factors associated with employment among people with severe mental illness. *The Journal of Nervous and Mental Disease*, 193, 705–713.

Sederer, L.I. & Clemens, N.A. (2003). The business case for high-quality mental health care. *Psychiatric Services*, 53, 143–145.

Slade E., & Salkever, D. (2001). Symptom effects on employment in a structural model of mental illness and treatment: analysis of patients with schizophrenia. *Journal of Mental Health Policy and Economics*, 4, 25–34.

Stapleton, D.C., O'Day, B.L., Livermore, G.A., & Imparato, A.J. (2006). Dismantling the poverty trap: disability policy for the twenty-first century. *Milbank Quarterly*, 84, 701–732.

Strauss, J.S. (2008). Is prognosis in the individual, the environment, the disease, or what? *Schizophrenia Bulletin*, 34, 245–246.

Tsang, H., Lam, P., Ng, B., & Leung, O. (2000). Predictors of employment outcome for people with psychiatric disabilities: a review of the literature since the mid '80's. *Journal of Rehabilitation*, 66, 19–25.

Velligan, D.I., Kern, R.S., & Gold, J.M. (2006). Cognitive rehabilitation for schizophrenia and the putative role of motivation and expectancies. *Schizophrenia Bulletin*, 32, 474–485.

Waghorn, G., & Lloyd, C. (2005). The employment of people with mental illness. *Australian e-Journal for the Advancement of Mental Health*, 4(2, Suppl.).

Wallace, C.J., & Tauber, R. (2004). Supplementing supported employment with workplace skills training. *Psychiatric Services*, 55, 513–515.

Wang, P.S., Beck, A.L., Berglund, P., McKenas, D.K., Pronk, N.P., Simon, G.E., & Kessler, R.C. (2004). Effects of major depression on moment-in-time work performance. *American Journal of Psychiatry*, 161, 1885–1891.

Wewiorski, N.J., & Fabian, E.S. (2004). Association between demographic and diagnostic factors and employment for people with psychiatric disabilities: a synthesis of recent research. *Mental Health Services Research*, 6, 9–21.

World Health Organization (2001). *International Classification of Function, Disability and Health*. Geneva: World Health Organization.

Chapter 12
SUPPORTED EDUCATION

Chris Lloyd and Samson Tse

Chapter overview

Many people with mental illness experience a disruption in their educational attainment, which often affects their employability. Supported education is a psychiatric rehabilitation intervention designed to assist people gain a valued role as a student and eventually a worker. This chapter addresses the health benefits of education, work delay, barriers to education, young people and mental illness, psychiatric rehabilitation and supported education, the Choose-get-keep programme model, characteristics predicting successful outcomes, and evaluation/outcomes. The chapter concludes by examining the features and strategies that practitioners can employ to develop supported education programmes.

Introduction

People with early-onset disability may have greater difficulties completing school. Lower educational attainment may in turn reduce the individual's employment and earning potential throughout his or her lifetime, leading people with early-onset disability to be doubly disadvantaged (Loprest & Maag, 2007). Having lower employment and earning potential can also lead to a greater likelihood of receiving disability pensions (Loprest & Maag, 2007). Loprest and Maag (2007) found that lower educational attainment resulted in employment rates being significantly lower than they would have been if education levels were comparable to those without disabilities. It is suggested that efforts to improve educational attainment should be an important part of efforts to increase employment for people with disabilities as increases in employment in the early years of a young person's life may have long-term positive effects, including greater accumulation of work experience and earnings.

Education and health benefits of education

According to Ross and Wu (1995), well-educated people experience better health than the poorly educated, as indicated by high levels of self-reported health and physical functioning and low levels of morbidity, mortality and disability. It has been reported that consumers of mental health services die on an average 25 years earlier than the general public (Everett et al., 2008). Well-educated people are less likely to be unemployed, and more likely to have full-time jobs, fulfilling work, high incomes and low economic hardship. Blustein (2008) suggested that work is critical to psychological health and well-being. People who are well educated are more likely to have social–psychological resources, including a high sense of personal control and social support (Cerin & Leslie, 2008). In addition, well-educated people are more likely to have healthier lifestyles in that they are more likely to exercise, to drink moderately, to receive preventive medical care and less likely to smoke (Cerin & Leslie, 2008; Ross & Wu, 1995). Education shapes work and economic conditions. It provides skills and information to help people cope with life stressors. Education is important in that occupations with greater prestige and status require a college education. Early career success may then set the tone for long-term success (Judge & Hurst, 2008).

Work delay

There are a number of possible correlates to work delay evident in the literature among people with mental illness. These include early application for disability pensions which discourages employment seeking (Kouzis & Eaton, 2000); restrained encouragement to seek work from mental health professionals (Baron & Salzer, 2000); and the fact that occupational functioning may be more influenced by cognitive disturbances to working memory than by the severity of symptoms (Barch, 2003). In a study conducted by Gioia (2006), she found that participants responded with themes of symptom severity and fear of symptoms on the job, medication side effects, disability benefits, family and cultural pressure, mental health professionals and advice about returning to work, ongoing parenting responsibilities and dependence on family and/or residential programmes; they were all factors contributing to work delay.

It is concerning that there is a lengthy delay in the return to work for many young adults after they are first diagnosed, and by not addressing this delay, a young adult may fall into a pattern of persistent non-employment. It can be seen that enhanced vocational approaches that emphasises the development and reliance on natural support networks and the pursuit of post-secondary education or vocational training would greatly benefit individuals who have psychiatric disabilities both personally and economically (Murphy et al., 2005).

Barriers to education

The impact of mental illness may be widespread with impairment in many psychosocial spheres, including occupational, interpersonal and marital areas, at times to the extent of affecting the person's ability to live independently in the community and pursue educational goals. Many people with severe mental illness experience their initial episodes in adolescence or young adulthood, thus eliminating or severely curtailing their opportunities for educational preparation and the acquisition of work skills, ethics and experiences (Fabian, 1999). There are a number of barriers which may impact upon young people being able to successfully complete their education. These may include:

- Symptoms of mental illness
- A lack of understanding or awareness of mental illness by faculty and peers
- Continuing stigma and discrimination
- Limited mental health service support/lack of resources
- Lack of support from family and/or mental health workers
- Financial problems
- Competing family responsibilities
- Side effects of medication, lack of confidence and worries about possible relapse (Mowbray et al., 1999, 2001a; Sasson et al., 2005)

External barriers were more likely to be reported by people with lower incomes and by those whose social networks were less supportive of educational goals. Personal barriers were more common among those who reported greater difficulty with psychiatric symptoms, greater substance abuse problems and lower overall quality of life. Programmatic barriers were more common among individuals who had previously attended college, who reported more symptomatology difficulties and whose social networks were less supportive of employment goals. Scheduling conflicts were more frequently expressed by people who had minor children, who were working prior to college enrolment, who attended their mental health programme less frequently and by people who were enrolled in college concurrently (Bybee et al., 2000). In an analysis of focus group data, Bybee et al. (2000) found barriers as being transportation difficulties, general financial problems, problems related to mental illness, scheduling conflicts, competing life problems and misunderstanding about the programme.

Government policies are pivotal in ensuring that mental health, the labour market, employment and income support policies work together to ensure progress towards participation in education by people with mental disability. For instance, in New Zealand, the Ministry of Health has responsibility for health policy advice, the District Health Boards for purchasing health and disability support services, some of which may have a pre-vocational component, and the education agencies for the provision of education and training programmes. The Department of Labour has responsibility for overall employment-related policy advice. Work and Income New Zealand (WINZ) provides employment placement and income support and funds a range of pre-vocational training and employment support services.

Such fragmentation of services may not be useful. It may be important to improve the integration of these different government departments. One change which aims at doing just this has been the transfer of responsibility for funding of vocational services from Children Young Persons and Their Families Agency to the WINZ, whose performance in this area is overseen by the Department of Labour within the Ministry of Social Development. The Department of Labour is also charged with funding the Workbridge organisation, an organisation that provides a specialist placement service for employers and people with all types of disability. Furthermore, the Training Incentive Grant is available from WINZ and training subsidies from Workbridge. These changes provide better alignment of each department's operational practices, which in turn should ensure better educational or pre-vocational services for people with mental illness.

Young people and mental illness

The onset of mental illness dramatically interrupts personal lives, often occurring during young adulthood when people are pursuing academic or vocational goals. Psychiatric symptoms and discriminatory treatment by others can start young people with mental illness on a downward course of educational underachievement or failure, underemployment or unemployment, and consequent lifelong disabilities (Bellamy & Mowbray, 1998; Mowbray et al., 1999). Young people with mental illness may experience a number of deficits including lacking in social resources, problems in interpersonal skills, and typically being unemployed (Anthony & Unger, 1991). They may also have a number of losses, which include personal losses due to serious mental illness and subjective losses related to symptoms and psychosocial losses due to changes in functioning and lack of access to valued social roles (Stein, 2005). Stein et al. (2005) studied the personal loss experienced by people with psychiatric disability. The results showed that these losses included the perceived loss of social roles and routines, loss of former relationships, loss of former self and loss of the future as a result of having a mental illness. Many of these young people have the desire, motivation and educational background to attend college (Bellamy & Mowbray, 1998).

Students with disabilities view access to post-secondary education as:

- An opportunity to enhance their chances of obtaining and maintaining employment
- A means of earning a higher annual income
- A pathway to lifelong independence and a greater quality of life (Bellamy & Mowbray, 1998; Wilson et al., 2000)

Rehabilitation practitioners have recognised that helping people restart their post-secondary educational pursuits is a desirable, valid and viable option.

Educational attainment is increasingly linked to meaningful employment and upward social mobility. In a study reported by Waghorn et al. (2004), it was found that higher education was positively associated with both employment and labour market participation.

Psychiatric rehabilitation and supported education

Psychiatric rehabilitation is strengths-based, focusing on the capabilities and competencies of people with psychiatric disabilities. The benefits of psychiatric rehabilitation are behavioural improvements and outcomes in the living, learning or working areas (Soydan, 2004). The two fundamental interventions of psychiatric rehabilitation are the development of skills and the development of environmental supports. Supported education helps people reclaim a valued role as a student, and eventually as a worker. This provides direct access to rehabilitation and in the process connects people with others. Soydan (2004) suggests that facilitating this phase of recovery are acceptance, coping skills, connecting sills, advocacy skills, opportunity for valued roles, risk taking, supported employment and education, and therapy. She believes that all of these activities and interventions are central in the process of returning to school.

Brockelman et al. (2006) conducted a postal survey in the US universities to investigate the relationship between sources of information and professors' perceptions of working with students with psychiatric disabilities. It was found that having had a friend with mental illness, knowing a student with mental illness and currently being on treatment for mental illness were strong predictors of professors' perceptions of and confidence in working with students with mental health problems. The descriptive findings also indicated that most of the professors who participated in the survey said that they did not have adequate knowledge or training to support students with mental illness and in some cases students did not always disclose their history of having diagnosed psychological disorder.

Supported education is defined as the provision of individualised, practical support and instruction to assist people with psychiatric disabilities to achieve their educational goals (Soydan, 2004). Supported education is tailored to meet the unique and changing needs of each student. Support and services are provided so that people with a severe mental illness can begin or continue post-secondary education. Mowbray (2004) lists the essential ingredients of supported education as being:

- Normalisation
- Self-determination
- Support and relationships
- Hope and recovery
- Systems change

Supported education helps students learn the skills, access the supports, and identify and use the academic adjustments necessary to successfully complete a class, course, degree or training program. Supported education provides access to the normalised environment of a campus and its potential for enhancing socialisation and interpersonal relationships, which results in the transformation of the self–image from patient to student (Frankie et al., 1996).

The major goals of supported education are:

- To improve post-secondary educational choice
- Access
- Retention through appropriate accommodations

Supported education addresses the following psychiatric rehabilitation objectives:

- Participation in normalising social and interpersonal environments
- Access to leisure, recreational and cultural resources available in educational settings
- Opportunities to strengthen basic educational competencies related to course requirements, e.g. study skills, time management
- Opportunities to develop individual interests related to career development and vocational choice
- Peer support
- Support to assist students to navigate the educational environment (Collins et al., 1998)

In order to assist students to navigate the educational environment or assist them to achieve the level of recovery ready for taking up formal, full-scale study, a variety of supported education initiatives have been implemented and evaluated. For example, in New Zealand, Clayton and Tse (2003) ran the 'health and well-being course' at local tertiary institution for people who had diagnosed mental illness and who were in recovery. The programme had two aims: (1) providing students with an opportunity to reflect and develop further skills for managing health and well-being and (2) encouraging students to participate more fully in their community such as opportunity for post-secondary education.

The pilot study consisted of nine students who had completed the 13-week-long part-time course (3 hours a day, 3 days a week) and consented to participate in the evaluation study. On the whole, students indicated a high level of satisfaction with the content and facilitation of the course. Out of the nine students, five enrolled in other post-secondary studies, which was a clear indication that students used the health and well-being course as a stepping stone to further education. Students' evaluations suggested two important features of the pilot programme. Firstly, students appreciated the fact that they were there as a student, not as a client. They were not expected to disclose a lot of their own personal issues or past experiences, but if they had personal issues, they could seek help from students support services. Secondly, according to the evaluation information, the pilot programme gave students an opportunity to pursue higher qualifications in an education environment, which was perceived by students as accepting and non-discriminatory (Clayton & Tse, 2003).

In Australia, Best et al. (2008) described a partnership between a college and a mental health service, which involved three supported education initiatives. The courses were horticulture, computing and hospitality. Sixty-one students participated in the programme since its inception. There were four key features that contributed to successful course completion. These were high levels of collaboration between staff at the two participating sites; teachers who were highly competent with delivering the course content and who had an understanding and empathy for disability; support provided was consistent across courses and mental health staff developed rapport with students that allayed any fears or misconceptions about college. The course completion rate was very close to the overall module completion rates for the general population (72% vs 77%).

Similarly, another supported education programme titled as 'Consumer as Provider' (CAP) was implemented and evaluated at the University of Kansas in the USA (Ratzlaff et al., 2006). The Kansas CAP programme which was a 15-week programme combining classroom learning and internship activities was set up to increase the educational pursuits and employability of consumers with a severe and persistent psychiatric disability. The CAP programme offered training as prerequisites for employment as case-management aides. One hundred fifty-seven students were accepted into the programme; 100 students graduated and 84 participated in the study and completed the survey questionnaires. The evaluation study of the CAP programme was thought to be the first study of its kind into investigating the effects of recovery training on participants or students' well-being. The results showed that CAP contributed to a significant increase in the participants' reported self-esteem and hope and an increase in the perception of recovery when using the retrospective measures. The simple pre–post design of Ratzlaff and colleagues' study limits their ability to attribute the results to the CAP programme. The research study did not report the 84 graduates' employment outcomes, but it mentioned approximately 60% of graduates were employed at 6-month and 2-year follow-up among the first batch of graduates.

Choose-get-keep programme model

The Choose-get-keep model focuses on a specific student and practitioner process using rehabilitation diagnostic, planning and intervention skills to guide the person to choose, get and keep an educational goal. The Choose-get-keep programme structure works to provide people with an opportunity to choose where they want to learn, and then to develop the skills and supports they need to be successful and satisfied as students (Soydan, 2004). The goal of choosing is to select an educational or training site compatible with the participant's values, skills, aptitudes, career interests, finances and learning objectives. The goal of getting is to secure enrolment in a preferred educational programme or training site. The goal of keeping is to sustain enrolment and maintain an acceptable level of success and satisfaction until completion/graduation (Soydan, 2004).

Choosing phase

The choosing phase is designed to assist people make an informed choice about where, when, why and how they want to attend school. An educational goal is the formulation of a statement of educational intent which specifies the student's preferred area of academic interest, school or training setting, number of classes per semester and target date for enrolment. A central part of the choosing phase is conducting a functional assessment and a resource assessment. A functional assessment provides a means for the supported education provider and the individual to develop an understanding of those skills the student can and cannot performrelated to achieving the educational goal. Skill areas might include competencies such as completing applications, organising work, taking notes, asking questions, asking for help, coping with stress, overcoming test anxiety, participating in group work with other students or improving concentration (Soydan, 2004). A resource assessment is also carried out. This measures the presence or absence of supports needed to meet the educational goal.

Getting phase

This phase is the planning section of the supported education process. Objectives are developed based on the assessment established in the choosing phase. Planning for successful enrolment involves negotiation of responsibility and scheduling times for completion of each of the tasks required to gain admission to a school. Useful skills for the student to gain in this phase include application completion, essay writing and bureaucracy management. During this phase it is important to identify and link with additional services that provide specific types of enrolment support such as financial aid. A final critical task during this phase is the identification of any needs for academic adjustments, for example allowing a student to bring in a tape recorder to the classroom, extended exam time. It may be necessary to look at administrative requirements, for example declaring part-time status, selecting classes or course load. It will be necessary to discuss the issue of disclosure of psychiatric disability in order to prepare any necessary disability documentation (Soydan, 2004).

Keeping phase

The keeping phase lasts the longest and involves the most time and energy commitment from both the student and practitioner. A wide range of skills may need to be taught. Skills specific to educational environments are useful in assessing levels of skill use, such as clarifying assignments, managing time, completing written assignments and preparing for tests. Resource development involves coordinating the link to resources so that it is available when needed. Support resources include tutors, advisors, counsellors, crisis intervention services and psychiatric services (Soydan, 2004).

Characteristics predicting successful outcomes

In a study conducted by Collins et al. (2000), it was found that no demographic characteristics were associated with productive activity at follow-up and that specific characteristics of mental illness, such as diagnosis, symptoms or length of illness, were not related to productive activity. Additional factors were that productive activity at baseline, financial resources and social supports were obtained. According to this research, among those with mental illness, social support is a key factor in attaining educational and vocational goals. Unger et al. (2000) found that the type of psychiatric diagnosis was not a predictor of school success but having one's own car and the number of psychiatric hospitalisations prior to programme participation were predictors. It was also found that the school retention rate was comparable to students without disability. Employment rates during the study were lower than other students but higher than the population of people with mental illness generally (Unger et al., 2000).

Evaluation/outcomes

In an evaluation/outcome of supported education initiative in London, Isenwater et al. (2002) found increase in self-esteem, social functioning, independence, cognitive abilities and confidence. In addition, some students reported that they felt less stigmatised with their problems and that their assertiveness had improved. There was a significant decrease in inpatient and day-patient hospitalisations. They suggest that peer support and support from lecturers were crucial factors in improving the student's self-esteem and functioning both within and outside of the college. Ponizovsky et al. (2004) in a study of supported education conducted in Israel found that students with a mental illness had higher distress scores than students without a disability; they used more emotion-oriented and avoidance-oriented coping strategies such as distraction and social diversion and the students had social support from family members and significant others but had a low level of social support. These findings suggest that it would be beneficial to have targeted specific interventions to enable students to prevent distress and to fully use the supported education programme, for example increase availability of social support, utilise more adaptive coping resources, and communications training, problem-solving and social skills training.

Ratzlaff et al. (2006) examined a student's perceptions of hope, self-esteem and recovery involved in the Consumer as Provider supported education programme. The findings showed involvement in the programme resulted in significantly increased levels of participant's hope and self-esteem. A student's level of recovery did not change significantly. In a qualitative study conducted by Knis-Matthews et al. (2007), participants diagnosed with a mental illness were interviewed to explore their experiences while attending a post-secondary school. Four main theses emerged from the interviews of the participants. These were education helped them to find a sense of purpose and transition into other life roles, the impact of mental illness made it difficult to stay consistent during their school years, their support systems and strategies contributed to their success at school and the supported education programme got them back into the classroom to see if they were ready to be a student again. They suggested that it was important that mental health providers and school administrators need to recognise that persons with mental illness can participate fully and successfully in a college setting with appropriate and reasonable accommodations, and that providing appropriate services to these students requires knowledge about their needs and concerns. Westwood (2003) conducted a qualitative research project examining the experience of attending an adult education course from the perspective of people with a mental illness. The results indicated that attending college improved confidence, self-esteem, socialisation and motivation. The participants gained knowledge and skills, had an increased purpose to the day and experienced improvements in their mental well-being.

Mowbray et al. (2001b) examined the needs, problems and satisfaction of participants in a supported education programme for adults with psychiatric disabilities. Participants were significantly satisfied with those items which were most central to college enrolment, such as applying for college and financial aid. The researchers suggested that in future programmes the following components should be included: support groups available, choosing a college major, more effective study habits, choosing a job and scheduling classes. Bybee et al. (2000) examined participation rates and self-reported barriers to attendance for adults with a mental illness who were participating in a supported education programme. The results indicated that women were more than four times as likely to participate, those who had had a job interview were less than one fifth as likely to participate, those who rated their residential quality of life higher were more likely to participate, and those with a more extensive social network and receiving more support for educational goals from one's social network were more likely to participate. Analysis of the focus group data showed that transportation, general financial problems, problems related to mental illness, scheduling problems, competing life problems and misunderstanding about the program were all mentioned as barriers to participation.

Features/strategies

In working with people who have a mental illness and who want to gain an education, there are a number of features about the campus that are important to consider when pursuing post-secondary education. This may include such things as:

- Is the campus atmosphere generally accepting of students with differences in learning styles and are they encouraged to participate fully in a variety of campus-life activities?
- Is there a specialised area of emphasis associated with the services?
- Are the school administration and faculty aware of the needs of students with disabilities?
- How are academic adjustments coordinated and are there specialised accommodations, e.g. note-takers?
- Is it possible to maintain a reduced course load and are extensions available?
- Is tutoring provided by peers or professional staff? (Wilson et al., 2000)

Sasson et al. (2005) suggest that an effective supported education programme includes three elements, namely formulation of policy, identification of the needs of the population and design, and implementation of the supported education programme. Policy provides a framework or mechanism to integrate health, education and other relevant services (e.g. incomes support, family support for those adults with young children) and investigates the needs for workforce training, for example training of the teaching staff, school principals, counsellors and rehabilitation practitioners who are specialised in working with young people. With regard to defining the needs of the population, it is paramount to identify who these young people are and what all is required to enable them pursue their educational opportunities. Waghorn et al. (2004) identified from the literature common features of supported education that appear to contribute to the effectiveness of supported education programmes. These features include the following:

- Coordinating across other services involving a person with mental illness to prevent other service providers disrupting the supported education programme
- Specialised staff are allocated to the supported education programmes and trained to specifically support educational objectives/goals

- Providing specialised career counselling, including vocational planning and exploration
- Assistance to access financial aid
- Skill building to cope with the academic environment
- On-campus information about student rights and resources
- On- or off-campus mentorship and support throughout the duration of the course
- Establish contacts within the educational institution to facilitate access to particular course and persons able to provide within-course assistance
- Access to tutoring, library assistance and other forms of supplemental educational support
- General support for the multiple individual barriers and life stressors which can lead to educational attrition

Conclusions

In our culture people want to work because they gain self-respect and dignity through work. People with a mental illness are not different. Young people with mental illness who are not in school or the workforce are doubly stigmatised. It seems that the most important factor affecting participation and level of employment activity is the amount of education completed. One of the goals of supported education is to improve career employment opportunities. Education is a valued entity in this society. It allows not only the opportunity to learn, but also the benefits related to it, such as employment and status and identity. Supported education is a promising method to improve the employment rates of people with psychiatric disability.

References

Anthony, W.A., & Unger, K.V. (1991). Supported education: an additional program resource for young adults with long term mental illness. *Community Mental Health Journal, 27,* 145–156.

Barch, D. (2003). Cognition in schizophrenia: does working memory work? *Current Directions in Psychological Science, 12,* 146–150.

Baron, R.C., & Salzer, M.S. (2000). The career patterns of persons with serious mental illness: generating a new vision of life time careers for those in recovery. *Psychiatric Rehabilitation Skills, 4,* 136–156.

Bellamy, C.D., & Mowbray, C.T. (1998). Supported education as an empowerment intervention for people with mental illness. *Journal of Community Psychology, 26,* 401–413.

Best, L.J., Still, M., & Cameron, G. (2008). Supported education: enabling course completion for people experiencing mental illness. *Australian Occupational Therapy Journal, 55,* 65–68.

Blustein, D.L. (2008). The role of work in psychological health and well-being. A conceptual, historical, and public policy perspective. *American Psychologist, 63*, 228–240.

Brockelman, K.F., Chadsey, J.G., & Loeb, J.W. (2006). Faculty perceptions of university students with psychiatric disabilities. *Psychiatric Rehabilitation Journal, 31*, 23–39.

Bybee, D., Bellamy, C., & Mowbray, C.T. (2000). Analysis of participation in an innovative psychiatric rehabilitation intervention: supported education. *Evaluation and Program Planning, 23*, 41–52.

Cerin, E., & Leslie, E. (2008). How socio-economic status contributes to participation in leisure-time physical activity. *Social Science and Medicine, 66*, 2596–2609.

Clayton, J., & Tse, S. (2003). An educational journey towards recovery for individuals with persistent mental illness: a New Zealand perspective. *Psychiatric Rehabilitation Journal, 27*, 72–78.

Collins, M.E., Bybee, D., & Mowbray, C.T. (1998). Effectiveness of supported education for individuals with psychiatric disabilities: results from an environmental study. *Community Mental Health Journal, 34*, 595–613.

Collins, M.E., Mowbray, C.T., & Bybee, D. (2000). Characteristics predicting successful outcomes of participants with severe mental illness in supported education. *Psychiatric Services, 51*, 774–780.

Everett, A., Mahler, J., Biblin, J., Ganguli, R., & Mauer, B. (2008). Improving the health of mental health consumers: effective policies and practices. *International Journal of Mental Health, 37*, 8–48.

Fabian, E.S. (1999). Rethinking work: the example of consumers with serious mental health disorders. *Rehabilitation Counselling Bulletin, 42*, 302–316.

Frankie, P.A., Levine, P., Mowbray, C.T., Shriner, W., Conklin, C., & Thomas, E.R. (1996). Supported education for persons with psychiatric disabilities: implementation in an urban setting. *Journal of Mental Health Administration, 23*, 406–417.

Gioia, D. (2006). Examining work delay in young adults with schizophrenia. *American Journal of Psychiatric Rehabilitation, 9*, 167–190.

Isenwater, W., Lanham, W., & Thornhill, H. (2002). The College Link Program: evaluation of a supported education initiative in Great Britain. *Psychiatric Rehabilitation Journal, 26*, 43–50.

Judge, T.A., & Hurst, C. (2008). How the rich (and happy) get richer (and happier): relationship of core self-evaluations to trajectories in attaining work success. *Journal of Applied Psychology, 93*, 849–863.

Knis-Matthews, L., Bokara, J., DeMeo, L., Lepore, N., & Mavus, L. (2007). The meaning of higher education for people diagnosed with a mental illness: four students share their experiences. *Psychiatric Rehabilitation Journal, 31*, 107–114.

Kouzis, A.C., & Eaton, W.W. (2000). Psychopathology and the initiation of disability payments. *Psychiatric Services, 51*, 908–913.

Loprest, P., & Maag, E. (2007). The relationship between earl disability onset and education and employment. *Journal of Vocational Rehabilitation, 26*, 49–62.

Mowbray, T. (2004). Supported education: diversity, essential ingredients, and future directions. *American Journal of Psychiatric Rehabilitation, 7*, 347–362.

Mowbray, C.T., Bellamy, C.D., Megivern, D., & Szilvagyi (2001a). Raising our sites: dissemination of supported education. *Journal of Behavioral Health Services and Research, 28*, 484–491.

Mowbray, C.T., Bybee, D., & Collins, M.E. (2001b). Follow-up client satisfaction in a supported education program. *Psychiatric Rehabilitation Journal, 24*, 237–247.

Mowbray, C.T., Collins, M., & Bybee, D. (1999). Supported education for individuals with psychiatric disabilities: long-term outcomes from an experimental study. *Social Work Research*, 23, 89–100.

Murphy, A.A., Mullen, M.G., & Spagnolo, A.B. (2005). Enhancing individual placement and support: promoting job tenure by integrating natural supports and supported education. *American Journal of Psychiatric Rehabilitation*, 8, 37–61.

Ponizovsky, A., Grinshpoon, A., Sasson, R., & Levav, I. (2004). Stress in adult students with schizophrenia in a supported education program. *Comprehensive Psychiatry*, 45, 401–407.

Ratzlaff, S., McDiarmid, D., Mary, D., & Rapp, C. (2006). The Kansas Consumer as Provider Program: measuring the effects of a supported education initiative. *Psychiatric Rehabilitation Journal*, 29, 174–182.

Ross, C.E., & Wu, C. (1995). The links between education and health. *American Sociological Review*, 60, 719–745.

Sasson, R., Grinspoon, A., Lachman, M., & Ponizovsky, A. (2005). A program of supported education for adult Israeli students with schizophrenia. *Psychiatric Rehabilitation Journal*, 29, 139–141.

Soydan, A.S. (2004). Supported education: a portrait of a psychiatric rehabilitation intervention. *American Journal of Psychiatric Rehabilitation*, 7, 227–248.

Stein, C.H. (2005). Aspirations, ability, and support: consumers' perceptions of attending college. *Community Mental Health Journal*, 41, 451–468.

Stein, C.H., Dworsky, D.O., Phillips, R.E., & Hunt, M.G. (2005). Measuring personal loss among adults coping with serious mental illness. *Community Mental Health Journal*, 41, 129–139.

Unger, K.V., Pardee, R., & Shafner, M. (2000). Outcomes of postsecondary supported education programs for people with psychiatric disabilities. *Journal of Vocational Rehabilitation*, 14, 195–199.

Waghorn, G., Still, M., Chant, D., & Whiteford, H. (2004). Specialised supported education for Australians with psychotic disorders. *Australian Journal of Social Issues*, 39, 443–458.

Westwood, J. (2003). The impact of adult education for mental health service users. *British Journal of Occupational Therapy*, 66, 505–510.

Wilson, K., Getzel, E., & Brown, T. (2000). Enhancing the post-secondary campus climate for students with disabilities. *Journal of Vocational Rehabilitation*, 14, 37–50.

Chapter 13

MANAGING PERSONAL INFORMATION IN SUPPORTED EMPLOYMENT FOR PEOPLE WITH MENTAL ILLNESS

Geoff Waghorn and Christine E. Spowart

Chapter overview

Employment specialists working with people with mental illness are aware of the potential for stigma and unfair discrimination when assisting clients with their competitive employment goals. However, few employment specialists develop explicit plans with clients to comprehensively manage their personal information in order to access reasonable accommodations while preventing stigma reactions and unfair discrimination in the workplace. A commonly used practice involves treating disclosure as a single binary decision presented to clients at programme entry. However, if clients choose non-disclosure, the subsequent range of employment services possible can be limited to behind the scenes assistance only, which can then impact adversely on employment outcomes attained. In this chapter we review stigma and disclosure evidence and suggest how an alternative strategy can be developed. We show how to plan the management of personal information while taking into account individual strengths, work restrictions and how these are best described and explained in the workplace and linked to an individual employment plan.

Introduction

Competitive employment is a feasible yet challenging goal for people with mental illness. Although some people manage to achieve employment goals without assistance, more encouraging employment outcomes are achieved by supported employment programmes designed specifically for people with severe mental illnesses. The most effective form of specialised supported employment is known as Individual Placement and Support (IPS), and has been more extensively investigated than other approaches in psychosocial rehabilitation (Bond, 2004; Bond et al., 2008). A recent review (Bond et al., 2008) shows that IPS services achieved competitive employment for 61% of clients compared to 23% among other vocational rehabilitation services. To our knowledge, no studies have examined disclosure strategies as possible reasons for some people failing to attain employment goals. This is surprising, given that disclosure strategies often determine the nature of employment assistance that can be provided.

Disclosure can also have costs and benefits (Corrigan & Matthews, 2003; Corrigan & Wassel, 2008). The costs include social avoidance and social disapproval, while the benefits include improved psychological well-being, improved interpersonal relationships and greater access to reasonable accommodations when needed (Fabian et al., 1993; MacDonald-Wilson et al., 2002). There is also emerging evidence that a planned-disclosure strategy leads to better workplace outcomes than an unplanned-disclosure strategy when a person suddenly becomes unwell (Ellison et al., 2003).

Employment specialists recognise the importance of planned disclosure as a means to obtain access to reasonable accommodations in the workplace and to prevent stigma and unfair discrimination (Tschopp et al., 2007). They also recognise the limitations of widely used alternative strategies such as concealment (Allen & Carlson, 2003) and recognise that the actual situations through which disclosure strategies must navigate can be complex (Goldberg et al., 2005). Hence, practical methods are needed to help employment specialists plan and implement more effective disclosure strategies. To date, these have not been developed, although some authors have suggested how this might be done (Hatchard, 2008; Harris et al., 2009; Waghorn et al., 2009a, b; Waghorn & Lewis, 2002). In addition, help with disclosure strategies is not yet recognised as part of evidence-based practices in supported employment (Bond, 2004).

Stigma and disclosure

Much has been written about stigma generally (Goffman, 1963) and how it applies to people with mental illness (Corrigan & Matthews, 2003; Rutman, 1994; World Health Organization, 2001). There are three main ways in which a person with mental illness can experience stigma: (1) through being unemployed and reliant on Government income support; (2) through mental illness diagnosis and treatment, or the consequences of mental illness; and (3) through a forensic or criminal history associated with the mental illness. Corrigan and Wassel (2008) identified three types of stigma that may act as barriers to life aspirations: public stigma, self-stigma and label avoidance. Although we know little about the best strategies to manage particular forms of stigma, it is clear that a more sophisticated approach is needed than simply treating disclosure as a binary (yes or no) decision at the point of entry to a supported employment programme (Waghorn & Lewis, 2002). (For more detailed information on stigma see Chapter 4.)

Stigma is known to hinder vocational recovery by impacting directly on the person and by reducing employment opportunities (Rutman, 1994; Waghorn & Lloyd, 2005). Some form of disclosure is also needed to access reasonable accommodations in the workplace. The provision of which has been linked to increased job tenure for people with mental illness (Fabian et al., 1993). Yet clients often prefer concealment to disclosure (Allen & Carlson, 2003), possibly because of prior negative experiences of stigma and fear of further unfair discrimination (Waghorn & Lewis, 2002). On the other hand, employment specialists may push clients toward partial or full disclosure to ensure that reasonable accommodations are accessible when needed. This push tendency may be driven by a fear of failure if disclosure is not permitted by the client. Hence, employment specialists and clients risk damaging their working alliance if a stable agreement on a suitable disclosure strategy is not achieved.

Anecdotal evidence suggests that many employment specialists find disclosure a complex and intimidating concept. Often they are instructed to simply give the client the choice and respect the client's choice, a choice which may not be revisited by either client or employment specialist again. Consequently, some employment specialists have caseloads in which the majority of clients have adopted a non-disclosure strategy. This in turn limits the service that can be provided, because it may preclude the employment specialist from contacting employers on the client's behalf. We also know that once clients have been given a choice and have adopted a non-disclosure strategy, it can be difficult to get them to agree to any form of disclosure to the employer, even when they become unwell. Furthermore, many employment specialists do not routinely ask clients about the reasons for their choice of disclosure strategy, and may not realise that initial strategies are often driven by past stigma experiences. For example, a client who has experienced stigma, shame and unfair discrimination in a workplace may prefer to avoid all forms of disclosure. Another client may have had repeated experiences of stigma whether they have disclosed or not, yet may insist on full disclosure as part of a personal advocacy effort to counter stigma in the wider community.

Normalising disclosure

In employment, disclosure may initially appear to be a simple problem of providing health and disability information to employers. In reality, disclosure is part of a complex ongoing process where the demand for potentially discrediting information emerges whenever new individuals and new situations are encountered. A fresh disclosure requirement can occur with each new supervisor appointed, with each change of duties or rosters and with each new co-worker allocated. Disclosure involves relabelling, reframing, filtering and customising information to fit a particular social context. These strategies can be particularly important to people with mental illness and represent methods of managing personal information. Whatever disclosure strategy is selected, including non-disclosure, the strategy needs to be consistent over time and needs to be effective in both formal and informal situations in the workplace (Waghorn & Lewis, 2002).

A recent qualitative study (Harris et al., 2009) has shown that from a client perspective, learning about disclosure strategies is important through implications of shame and embarrassment if disclosure is poorly managed. We sought to normalise disclosure by examining what people do when they do not have any particular need for a disclosure strategy. The equivalent strategy in use by healthy job seekers is to manage their personal information by preparing a personal resume to summarise the information that prospective employers want to know while concealing less favourable information. This is the aim of every resume or curriculum vitae to manage personal information by presenting a favourable summary of the person and their work history tailored to job requirements.

The main difference for people with mental illness is the extent of the challenge. The personal information to be managed can be more damaging to their employment prospects and, therefore, must be managed more carefully. However, too much focus on disclosure of negative information distracts clients from their own strengths and resources, and may also trigger negative emotions associated with memories of negative stigma experiences. Therefore, we think a better way is needed to help clients solve the disclosure dilemma. We considered Hatchard's (2008) approach to disclosure based on a concept of occupational competence. However, we think we can improve on this by viewing disclosure in the same way as workers without health conditions, which also allows clients to reduce their self-stigma. This involves developing a comprehensive plan to manage the full range of relevant personal information including a person's individual strengths. Initial feedback from clients is that this approach is empowering because new choices are provided, whereas previously they did not exist or were made by the employment specialist. The process of jointly developing a personal information management plan was also perceived as a normalising experience because the term 'disclosure' was not used and the plan did not focus too much on the problem of sharing potentially discrediting information.

Developing a plan to manage personal information

We considered the steps involved in developing a successful plan. A personal information plan is best developed at programme entry soon after vocational goals are identified and a suitable short list of candidate jobs are identified for job tryouts. A single sheet plan format was considered essential because it needs to seem familiar, through being similar to how employment specialists already develop individual employment plans. We suggested that the two plans are coordinated by transferring the employment goal to the personal information plan, and by not repeating strengths in the personal information plan if these are already noted in the individual employment plan. Instead, the focus can shift to more specific examples of strengths in terms of knowledge, skills, attitudes and resources that can help offset any negative emotional consequences from identifying specific work restrictions. The first column of the plan records the vocational goals or specific jobs for tryouts listed in the individual employment plan. The following sections discuss how the remaining six columns of the plan can be completed collaboratively during an interview with the client (see Table 13.1).

A strengths-based approach (column 2)

A strengths-based approach (Marty et al., 2001; Rapp et al., 2005) is needed early in the plan to focus on information about the person's employment-related strengths. In this stage the focus can be on the personal characteristics that the employer might value that would help the person become a productive worker in that particular job or industry. It may take some time and patience for the employment specialist to elicit information about particular strengths from the client because self-stigma, low expectations, lack of a recent work history and low work confidence may cause people to think that they don't have anything of value to offer to employers. A strengths-based approach can be used to discuss the following with clients: (1) previous relevant employment experiences, (2) relevant knowledge, (3) relevant skills, (4) relevant attitudes and (5) resources available to the client to help manage their health and personal circumstances. Examples of these can be listed in the plan as strengths with respect to the client's current employment goal.

Identifying sensitive information (column 3)

The purpose of this column is to record the diagnostic terms, custodial periods and historical information that are potentially discrediting and need to be well managed. This is the first step in a systematic process covered by columns 3–5. The client's own words should be captured as much as possible, yet important information known by the employment specialist should also be suggested to the client for inclusion at this point. The descriptors identified in this column are not intended for further use. The second goal of this section is to help the employment specialist understand the client's prior stigma experiences and prior disclosure methods so that the reasons for specific pieces of information being considered sensitive are understood. One way to initiate this discussion is to ask clients about their past and present experiences of stigma, what they did in response to those experiences and how those experiences might influence their current thinking about how to manage personal information. A key question is: How was that piece of personal information managed previously and did that method contribute to the stigma or unfair discrimination experience?

Table 13.1 A sample plan to manage personal information.

Vocational goals, jobs, or employers of interest	Personal strengths	Sensitive information	Associated barriers or work restrictions	Agreed terms to describe and explain work restrictions in both formal and informal situations	Terms for use by client, employment specialist, supervisor	Workplace assistance or accommodations that may be needed
Gain employment in retail industry	Certificate II in Retail operations Customer service Hardworking Committed Motivated	Mental illness, schizophrenia	Attention and concentration Disorganised thoughts and activities do not always follow routines	Formal: Difficulty with attention on one task for extended periods Informal: Become bored easily when doing repetitive tasks Formal: Difficulty planning and organising tasks Informal: Sometimes loses track of priorities	Client, employment specialist	Requires diverse range of duties to remain task focused Additional assistance with planning tasks, priorities and time management

Client signature _____ Date _____

Employment specialist signature _____ Date _____

Plan to be next reviewed on Date _____

Identifying work barriers or work restrictions (column 4)

The aim of this column is to reframe or relabel diagnostic terms as descriptors of work restrictions using terms that employers and co-workers will understand. The idea is to identify specific ways in which each health condition produces limitations to employment in a particular job or industry, in terms of hours worked, type of duties or any other relevant information. Visible signs of illness should be accounted for and information about strengths can also be identified that can be added to this column to maintain the balance of positive and negative information. If no visible signs of illness are present, there is a greater opportunity to select terms that enable work performance strengths and need for assistance to be discussed with employers.

Employment specialists are aware of the negative effects of a variety of mental health labels in job applications, resumes and job interviews. Some labels have less negative effects than others. The term 'mental health problem' is more acceptable to employers than 'severe mental illness' or 'schizophrenia' (Waghorn & Lewis, 2002). However, a better approach is to avoid mental health terms altogether or use the generic term 'health condition'. Almost all medical and psychiatric terms can be reframed into work-related terms that shift the focus from the diagnostic category to specific work restrictions in a particular job. Most employment specialists know how to do this for particular individuals in specific work settings. For example, if the most relevant feature of a person's schizophrenia is the disorganised syndrome, the person can be described to the employer as 'having difficulty in planning and organising tasks'.

How terms will be used (columns 5–6)

Once terms describing work restrictions have been identified, how these terms are best used can then be discussed. The aim is to reach an agreement on who will use what terms and in what situations. Both formal (job applications, job interviews, meetings with supervisors and co-workers) and informal situations (lunchroom, casual conversations with co-workers) need to be considered. It is important to empower clients to decide exactly what terms the employment specialist can use when contacting employers on the client's behalf, in general service activities, and in discussions with other employment service staff and other organisations. Terms and their conditions for use can be specified in this column.

Accommodations or assistance needed (column 7)

Accommodations that may be needed can be discussed in terms of what may be needed in this job now during the training phase, and what may be needed later if the person becomes more unwell. It is possible that good job selection and identification of suitable hours of employment may be all that is required for now. Aspects of job redesign, workplace accommodations, additional on-site training, aids or equipment can all be considered. Information can be added to this column at regular intervals as the client and the employment specialist become aware of accommodations and forms of assistance that help to improve work performance. Just because items are identified here does not mean these are to be discussed with the employer. Increasing client control over their personal information and how it is used is fundamental to the purpose of the plan. Therefore, how and when these items are best raised with the employer can be specified, so that both parties are clear about how this information will be used.

Challenges facing employment specialists

Employment specialists will need to reconceptualise disclosure from a simple binary decision to a more fluid ongoing concept about how to manage information that will challenge both themselves and the client at different times and in different ways. 'Personal information' is a normalising term, something everyone has and have to manage, whereas 'disclosure' implies shame and guilt and involves a high risk for the client by the sudden exposure of sensitive information that may not be correctly understood by the people receiving the information. A plan to manage personal information puts disclosure in its proper context and enables any negative information to be offset by information about strengths.

Without a plan to manage personal information, many employment specialists may perceive the disclosure process as too difficult to discuss with clients in detail. When the disclosure dilemma is raised with clients, these questions follow: When should I disclose? What should I say? What should I say about my work restrictions? What are the implications of disclosure? Employment specialists expect that if clients have had any negative disclosure experiences then that will be something they would want to avoid.

Developing a personal information management plan avoids the problems created by conceptualising disclosure as a single binary decision. The new approach allows the client and the employment specialist to develop a stronger working alliance through creating a strategic plan that is strength focused and which describes how client confidentiality and privacy will be respected. The plan can also transfer skills to the clients, particularly in terms of how to manage their information in informal settings. This in turn is expected to increase client empowerment and confidence in the workplace, and reduce the risk of job loss through the shame of personal information being disclosed without permission. One way to check that the plan is developed along these lines is to see that how often the word disclosure is used. It is intended that the word not be used in any part of the plan, except perhaps with respect to past stigma experiences and identifying sensitive information.

Although the utility of this new approach in supported employment has not yet been established, a plan was developed and tested with a client prior to attending a job interview with promising results. This client had previously disclosed to some employers via their employment specialist but was unsure if the information was given to employers appropriately because no records were kept. The client completed the new plan with assistance from the employment specialist and then a mock interview was conducted to allow the client to practice using the terms chosen. The client reported feeling empowered by the approach and its specificity as well as feeling confident in the information selected for use in the workplace. The client has since reported being offered a position as a result of the job interview.

Conclusions

Through re-examining the evidence on stigma and disclosure we have developed a more practical way to manage personal information to minimise the risk of stigma and unfair discrimination in the workplace. We aimed to increase client empowerment and put clients back in control of decisions about how their personal information is to be managed throughout their careers. The result is a proposed method with substantial face validity and congruence with the evidence on how stigma impacts on the employment aspirations of people with mental illness. While this approach seems an improvement over offering clients a binary choice about disclosure, its reliability, utility and predictive validity in supported employment are yet to be established. Nevertheless, we see this as a promising step forward and encourage other researchers to study whether new methods such as this can improve employment outcomes for people with mental illness.

References

Allen, S. & Carlson, G. (2003). To conceal or disclose a disabling condition? A dilemma of employment transition. *Journal of Vocational Rehabilitation*, 19, 19–30.

Bond, G.R. (2004). Supported employment: evidence for an evidence-based practice. *Psychiatric Rehabilitation Journal*, 27, 345–359.

Bond, G.R., Drake, R.E., & Becker, D.R. (2008). An update on randomized controlled trials of evidence-based supported employment. *Psychiatric Rehabilitation Journal*, 31, 280–290.

Corrigan, P.W., & Matthews, A.K. (2003). Stigma and disclosure: implications for coming out of the closet. *Journal of Mental Health*, 12, 235–248.

Corrigan, P.W., & Wassel, A. (2008). Understanding and influencing the stigma of mental illness. *Journal of Psychosocial Nursing and Mental Health Services*, 46, 42–48.

Ellison, M.L., Russinova, Z., MacDonald-Wilson, K.L., & Lyass, A. (2003). Patterns and correlates of workplace disclosure among professionals and managers with psychiatric conditions. *Journal of Vocational Rehabilitation*, 18, 3–13.

Fabian, E.S., Waterworth, A., & Ripke, B. (1993). Reasonable accommodations for workers with serious mental illness: type, frequency, and associated outcomes. *Psychosocial Rehabilitation Journal, 17,* 163–172.

Goffman, E. (1963). *Stigma. Notes on the Management of Spoiled Identity.* Ringwood, VIC, Australia: Penguin.

Goldberg, S.G., Killeen, M.B., & O'Day, B. (2005). The disclosure conundrum: how people with psychiatric disabilities navigate employment? *Psychology, Public Policy, and Law, 11,* 463–500.

Harris, M., Cleary, C., King, J., & Waghorn, G. (2009). Development and preliminary evaluation of an employment resource for mental health service consumers, carers, and clinicians. *Australian e-journal for the Advancement of Mental Health, 8*(1), 1–15.

Hatchard, K. (2008). Disclosure of mental health. *Work, 30,* 311–316.

MacDonald-Wilson, K.L., Rogers, E.S., Massaro, J.M., Lyass, A., & Crean, T. (2002). An investigation of reasonable workplace accommodations for people with psychiatric disabilities: quantitative findings from a multi-site study. *Community Mental Health Journal, 38,* 35–50.

Marty, D., Rapp, C.A., & Carlson, L. (2001). The experts speak: the critical ingredients of strengths model case management. *Psychiatric Rehabilitation Journal, 24,* 214–221.

Rapp, C., Saleeby, D., & Sullivan, W.P. (2005). The future of strengths-based social work. *Advances in Social Work, 6,* 79–90.

Rutman, I.D. (1994). How psychiatric disability expresses itself as a barrier to employment. *Psychosocial Rehabilitation Journal, 17,* 15–35.

Tschopp, M.K., Perkins, D.V., Hart-Katuin, C., Born, D.L., & Holt, S.L. (2007). Employment barriers and strategies for individuals with psychiatric disabilities and criminal histories. *Journal of Vocational Rehabilitation, 26,* 175–187.

Waghorn, G., Chant, D., Lloyd, C., & Harris, M. (2009a). Labour market conditions, labour force activity, and prevalence of psychiatric disorders. *Social Psychiatry and Psychiatric Epidemiology, 44,* 171–178.

Waghorn, G., & Lewis, S. (2002). Disclosure of psychiatric disabilities in vocational rehabilitation. *Australian Journal of Rehabilitation Counselling, 8,* 67–80.

Waghorn, G., & Lloyd, C. (2005). The employment of people with mental illness. *Australian e-Journal for the Advancement of Mental Health, 4*(2, Suppl.), 1–43.

Waghorn, G., Harris, M., King, J., Cleary, C., & Lloyd, C. (2009b). *Building a Career of Your Choice: A Guide for Service Users, Families, and Mental Health Professionals.* Canberra: Mental Health Branch, Department of Health and Ageing.

World Health Organization (2001). *The World Health Report 2001 – Mental Health: New Understanding, New Hope.* Geneva: World Health Organization.

INDEX